CKD STAGE 4

COOKBOOK

Nourishing Your Body and Supporting Kidney Health with Low Potassium, Low Sodium, and Low Phosphorus Meals with 30-Day Meal Plan

Dr Brenda White

Copyright ©Brenda White, 2024.

All rights reserved. No part of this publication may be reproduced, distributed, or transmitted in any form or by any means, including photocopying, recording, or other electronic or mechanical methods, without the prior written permission of the publisher, except for brief quotations embodied in critical reviews and specific other non-commercial uses permitted by copyright law.

Table of Contents

Introduction 8
- Stages of CKD 9
- Signs and Symptoms 9
- Causes 10
- Risk Factors 11
- Complications 11
- Prevention 12
- Ten ways to manage kidney disease 12
- What If My Kidneys Fail? 13
- Treatment Options 13
- Kidney Disease in Children 13
- What are the signs of kidney disease in kids? 14
- What causes kidney disease in kids? 15

Living with CKD Stage 4 16
- Symptoms of stage 4 kidney disease 16
- Seeing a doctor when you have stage 4 CKD 16
- Treatment options for those in stage 4 17
- Diet and stage 4 CKD 17
- Medications and stage 4 CKD 17

Building a CKD-Friendly Pantry 18
- Food to Include and Avoid 18
- Substitution Tips 20
- Tips for making healthy food choices 23

Meal Planning 24
Breakfast Recipes 30
Lunch Recipes 40
Dinner Recipes 50
Snacks and Appetizers 60
Desserts 70
Beverages 82

Chapter 8: Special Diet Considerations 90
Diabetic-Friendly Recipes 90
Low-Sodium Recipes for Hypertension 103
Vegetarian CKD Recipes 114

Practical Tips and Resources 128
Cooking Techniques for CKD 128

Conclusion 132

Introduction

Chronic kidney disease, often referred to as chronic kidney failure, is characterized by the kidneys gradually losing their ability to function properly. The main job of the kidneys is to cleanse the blood by filtering out waste and excess fluid, which is then expelled from the body in urine. When the disease reaches an advanced stage, it can lead to harmful accumulations of fluid, electrolytes, and waste in the body.

In its initial stages, chronic kidney disease may not cause any noticeable symptoms, making it possible for someone to have the disease without being aware of it until it's quite advanced.

Managing chronic kidney disease involves trying to slow down the damage to the kidneys, typically by addressing the underlying cause. However, even with proper management, the disease can continue to progress. In its most severe form, chronic kidney disease can lead to end-stage kidney failure, which can be life-threatening if not treated with dialysis or a kidney transplant.

In the United States, around 37 million people, or 15% of the population, are affected by chronic kidney disease. It often remains unnoticed and undiagnosed until it has significantly progressed.

Certain ethnic groups, including African Americans, Hispanics, Native Americans, and Asian Americans, are at a higher risk of developing chronic kidney disease compared to white individuals, possibly due to healthcare disparities.

As kidney disease progresses, waste can accumulate quickly in the body. The goal of treatment is to halt or slow down the worsening of kidney function by managing the root cause.

Stages of CKD

Stage 1: A person with stage 1 chronic kidney disease has a GFR (glomerular filtration rate) of 90 ml/min per 1.73 m2 or higher, indicating normal kidney function but with signs of kidney damage, such as protein in the urine or physical damage to the kidneys.

Stage 2: At this stage, the GFR is between 60 and 89 ml/min per 1.73 m2. While this suggests the kidneys are still functioning well, there are additional indications of kidney damage.

Stage 3: This stage is split into two sub-stages:

- **Stage 3a:** With a GFR of 45–59 ml/min per 1.73 m2.
- **Stage 3b:** With a GFR of 30–44 ml/min per 1.73 m2.

Symptoms might include swelling in hands and feet, back pain, more frequent urination, anemia, high blood pressure, and bone disease.

People with stages 1 to 3 can potentially slow kidney damage by controlling blood sugar and blood pressure, eating healthily, avoiding tobacco, staying active, keeping a moderate weight, and consulting with a kidney specialist.

Stage 4: Here, the GFR drops to 15–29 ml/min per 1.73 m2, indicating moderate to severe kidney damage. It's a critical stage that precedes kidney failure, and symptoms and complications become more common.

Stage 5: This final stage is characterized by a GFR of less than 15 ml/min per 1.73 m2, meaning the kidneys are failing or close to it. Symptoms of kidney failure include itching, muscle cramps, nausea, vomiting, swelling, back pain, frequent urination, sleep difficulties, and trouble breathing. Treatment at this stage requires dialysis or a kidney transplant to help filter the blood since the kidneys can no longer do so effectively.

Signs and Symptoms

As chronic kidney disease progresses gradually, the signs and symptoms may take time to appear. The slow deterioration of kidney function can lead to the accumulation of fluids, waste, and imbalances in electrolytes. The severity of kidney function loss can lead to various issues, such as:

- Feeling nauseous
- Throwing up
- A decrease in hunger
- Tiredness and a lack of energy

- Trouble sleeping
- Changes in how often you pee
- Less mental clarity
- High blood pressure that resists treatment
- Breathlessness if fluid accumulates in the lungs
- Chest discomfort if fluid surrounds the heart
- Puffiness around the eyes
- Swollen legs
- Persistent breathlessness
- Unintentional weight reduction
- Breath that smells like urine
- Tingling in your hands and feet
- Easy bruising or bleeding
- Pain in the bones
- Alterations in skin, hair, or nails
- Feeling sleepy or mentally foggy
- Problems with sexual function
- Persistent itching
- Muscle spasms and cramps
- Blood in your stool
- Persistent hiccups
- Excessive thirst
- Reduced sexual interest

Causes

Several diseases and conditions can lead to chronic kidney disease, including:

- Diabetes (both type 1 and type 2)
- Persistent high blood pressure
- Glomerulonephritis, which is swelling of the kidney's filters
- Interstitial nephritis, which is inflammation of the kidney's tubules and surrounding areas
- Hereditary kidney conditions like polycystic kidney disease
- Long-term blockage of the urinary tract from conditions like enlarged prostate, kidney stones, or some cancers
- Vesicoureteral reflux, a condition causing urine to back up into your kidneys

- Repeated kidney infections

Risk Factors

Several factors can raise your chances of developing chronic kidney disease:

- Diabetes
- High blood pressure
- Cardiovascular disease
- Smoking
- Excess weight
- Ethnic backgrounds such as Black, Native American, or Asian American
- A family history of kidney issues
- Abnormal kidney structure
- Advancing age
- Regular use of medications that may harm the kidneys
- Cigarette use
- High cholesterol levels
- Autoimmune diseases
- Obstructive kidney disease, including complications from benign prostatic hyperplasia
- Atherosclerosis
- Liver conditions like cirrhosis
- Narrowing of the kidney-supplying artery
- Kidney or bladder cancer
- Kidney stones or infections
- Conditions like systemic lupus erythematosus
- Diseases like scleroderma or vasculitis
- Vesicoureteral reflux, where urine flows backward into the kidney

Complications

Kidney disease can have a wide-ranging impact on your body. Here are some issues it might cause:

- Swelling in your limbs and high blood pressure due to fluid buildup, or even fluid in your lungs
- Dangerous spikes in your blood's potassium levels, which can mess with your heart and be serious.
- Anemia, which means your blood doesn't have enough red cells

- Heart problems
- Weaker bones and a higher chance of breaking them
- A drop in your sex drive, trouble with getting an erection, or fertility issues
- Brain and nerve issues that can lead to trouble focusing, personality shifts, or seizures
- A weaker immune system, making you more prone to catching bugs
- Inflammation around your heart called pericarditis
- Risks during pregnancy for both mom and baby
- Kidney failure that's so bad you might need dialysis or a new kidney to stay alive

Prevention

- **Be smart with over-the-counter meds:** Stick to the recommended doses for things like aspirin, ibuprofen, and acetaminophen to avoid hurting your kidneys.
- **Keep your weight in a healthy range:** Stay active to maintain or get to a weight that's good for you.
- **Quit smoking:** It's bad news for your kidneys, and if you need a hand stopping, there's help there from support groups to meds.
- Team up with your doctor to manage any conditions that could hurt your kidneys.

Ten ways to manage kidney disease

- Keep your blood pressure in check
- If you've got diabetes, manage your blood sugar
- Regularly check your kidney health with your healthcare team
- Take your meds as they're prescribed
- Plan your meals with a dietitian's help
- Make exercise a regular thing
- Aim for a healthy weight
- Get plenty of sleep
- Stop smoking
- Find good ways to deal with stress and feeling down

What If My Kidneys Fail?

While some individuals manage to live with kidney disease for many years and keep their kidney function stable, others may experience a rapid decline leading to kidney failure.

Kidney failure occurs when the kidneys can no longer perform their duties effectively, operating at less than 15 percent of their normal capacity. At this stage, waste products and excess fluid may accumulate in the body, potentially causing various symptoms.

To replace your lost kidney function, you may have one of three treatment options:

- Hemodialysis
- Peritoneal dialysis
- Kidney transplant
- Managing end-stage renal disease (ESRD) with dialysis or a transplant

Some kids with kidney failure might opt out of dialysis or transplantation and instead focus on managing their condition with the support of their healthcare team, medications, and careful attention to diet and lifestyle.

Treatment Options

The treatment for chronic kidney disease (CKD) depends on its severity.

The primary approaches include:

- Lifestyle modifications to keep as healthy as possible
- Medications to address problems like high blood pressure and cholesterol
- Dialysis to mimic kidney function, often needed in stage 5 CKD
- Kidney transplant, which might be necessary for stage 5 CKD

Kidney Disease in Children

How often does kidney disease occur in kids?

Kidney disease isn't very common in children, and it's hard to pinpoint the exact number affected since many don't show symptoms in the early stages.

Which kids are more likely to get kidney disease?

Boys are more likely to have CKD than girls. In North America, Black children face a two to three times higher risk of developing CKD compared to white children.

What complications can arise from kidney disease in kids?

Some of the complications include:

- Anemia
- Heart disease
- Imbalances in blood electrolytes, like potassium
- Growth issues, such as being shorter than average
- High blood pressure
- Infections
- Metabolic acidosis
- Mineral and bone disorders
- Cognitive difficulties
- Urinary incontinence

What are the signs of kidney disease in kids?

Early-stage kidney disease might not cause any symptoms in children. But as it progresses, the signs can include:

- Swelling in the feet, legs, hands, or face (edema)
- Changes in urine output, possibly needing to pee more often or bedwetting
- Foamy urine from excess protein (proteinuria)
- Pink or cola-colored urine due to blood presence (hematuria)

Other possible symptoms are:

- Decreased appetite
- Fatigue
- Fevers
- High blood pressure
- Itchy skin
- Nausea or vomiting
- Shortness of breath
- Difficulty concentrating
- Weakness
- Weight loss
- Stunted growth

These symptoms can vary based on the underlying cause of the kidney disease.

What causes kidney disease in kids?

Kidney disease in children can result from:

- Birth defects
- Genetic conditions
- Infections
- Nephrotic syndrome
- Systemic diseases
- Trauma
- Urinary blockages or reflux

Living with CKD Stage 4

Individuals with stage 4 chronic kidney disease have experienced significant kidney impairment, with their glomerular filtration rate (GFR) dropping to a range between 15 and 30 ml/min. At this advanced stage, it's common for patients to be on the cusp of requiring dialysis or considering a kidney transplant.

As the kidneys fail to filter waste efficiently, toxins accumulate in the bloodstream, leading to a condition called uremia. Stage 4 also brings a higher risk of developing other health issues like hypertension, anemia, bone disorders, and cardiovascular diseases.

Symptoms of stage 4 kidney disease

- Tiredness
- Swelling due to fluid retention, particularly in the limbs, along with breathing difficulties
- Changes in urine, such as a foamy appearance, abnormal colors (like dark orange, brown, or red if blood is present), and alterations in frequency
- Pain in the back where the kidneys are located
- Disrupted sleep caused by muscle cramps or restless legs
- Feelings of nausea or vomiting
- A persistent metallic taste in the mouth
- Bad breath because of urea accumulation
- Decreased appetite, which may be accompanied by changes in taste or bad breath
- Difficulty focusing on daily tasks
- Nerve issues, such as numbness or tingling in the extremities

Seeing a doctor when you have stage 4 CKD

Regular check-ups with a nephrologist are essential at this stage. These kidney specialists conduct thorough examinations and order lab tests every three months or so to tailor the treatment plan, which might include preparing for dialysis or a transplant.

Treatment options for those in stage 4

1. **Hemodialysis:** This can be performed at a center or home with a partner's help, using a machine to filter blood.
2. **Peritoneal dialysis:** a needle-free option that can be done at home or even at work without a care partner.
3. **A kidney transplant:** often the most desired option, which comes with fewer dietary restrictions compared to dialysis.

Diet and stage 4 CKD

- Reducing protein intake to decrease waste buildup
- Including certain grains, fruits, and vegetables, assuming potassium and phosphorus levels are stable
- Limiting phosphorus to maintain normal PTH levels, prevent bone disease, and possibly preserve kidney function
- Restricting potassium if levels are elevated
- Moderating calcium intake
- Reducing carbohydrate consumption for diabetic patients
- Cutting back on saturated fats to manage cholesterol levels
- Lowering sodium intake, especially for those with high blood pressure or fluid issues
- Adjusting calcium intake according to blood levels
- Taking specific water-soluble vitamins like vitamin C and B complex, avoiding over-the-counter supplements unless approved by the nephrologist

Medications and stage 4 CKD

Medication adherence is crucial for managing blood pressure and blood sugar levels, which can help prolong kidney function.

Lifestyle choices are also important. Regular exercise and avoiding smoking can contribute to better health outcomes. Patients should consult their doctors for an appropriate exercise regimen and support with smoking cessation.

Building a CKD-Friendly Pantry

Food to Include and Avoid

Foods Containing More Sodium:

- Processed meats such as bacon, corned beef, ham, hot dogs, luncheon meats, and sausages
- Condensed and instant soups, bouillon cubes, and ramen noodle packs
- Pre-packaged mixes for dishes like hamburgers and pancakes
- Preserved vegetables, vegetable juices, and canned beans, chicken, fish, and meats
- Tomato-based products such as canned tomatoes and tomato juice
- Cottage cheese
- Frozen prepared meals
- Vegetables with added sauces in frozen form
- Pickled items including olives, pickles, and relishes
- Snack foods like pretzels, chips, crackers, and salted nuts
- Boxed meals and side dishes that are ready to eat
- Dressings for salads, bottled condiments, and marinades
- Salt and flavored salts like garlic salt
- Pre-mixed seasonings and sauce packets
- Certain ready-to-eat cereals, baked goods, and bread
- Soy sauce

Foods Containing Less Sodium:

- Popcorn made by air-popping
- Cooked cereals without any added salt
- Fresh cuts of meat, poultry, and seafood
- Fresh or frozen produce
- Frozen dinners, peanut butter, and salad dressings with reduced sodium
- Cheeses that are low in fat and sodium
- Rice and noodles without added salt
- Nuts that are not salted

Foods With Higher Potassium Content:

- Various fruits such as fresh apricots, bananas, cantaloupe, dates, kiwi, nectarines, oranges and their juice, prunes and prune juice, raisins
- An array of vegetables including acorn and butternut squash, avocados, baked beans, various greens like beets, cooked broccoli, cooked brussels sprouts, chard, chili peppers, cooked mushrooms, potatoes, pumpkin, cooked spinach, legumes such as split peas, lentils, and beans, sweet potatoes and yams, tomatoes in various forms such as juice and sauce, and vegetable juice

Foods With Lower Potassium Content:

- Fruits like apples and their juice, canned apricots and apricot nectar, various berries, cranberry juice, fruit cocktails, grapefruit, grapes and grape juice, lemons, limes, papayas, peaches, pears, pineapple, plums, rhubarb, tangerines, watermelon
- Vegetables such as alfalfa sprouts, canned bamboo shoots, bell peppers, fresh broccoli, cabbage, carrots, cauliflower, raw celery and onions, corn, cucumber, eggplant, green beans, kale, lettuce, fresh mushrooms, okra, cooked summer squash

Foods Rich in Phosphorus:

- Legumes like beans, lentils, nuts
- Bran cereals and oatmeal
- Certain beverages such as cola and some bottled iced teas
- Dairy products including milk, cheese, and yogurt
- Ice cream
- Processed meats like hot dogs and canned meats

Foods Low in Phosphorus:

- Corn and rice-based cereals
- A variety of fresh fruits and vegetables
- Home-brewed iced tea
- Rice milk that is not enriched
- Sorbet
- Meats that are not processed

Substitution Tips

Protein Substitutions

High-Phosphorus or High-Potassium Proteins

- **Substitute Red Meat** (beef, pork) with:
  - **Skinless Chicken Breast**: Lower in phosphorus and potassium.
  - **Fish** (like cod or tilapia): Lower in phosphorus and provides healthy omega-3 fatty acids.
  - **Tofu**: A versatile, plant-based protein that's kidney-friendly when prepared properly.

Dairy Products

- **Substitute Whole Milk** with:
  - **Unsweetened Almond Milk**: Lower in potassium and phosphorus.
  - **Rice Milk**: Another low-potassium and low-phosphorus option.

Cheese

- **Substitute High-Phosphorus Cheeses** (like cheddar) with:
  - **Low-sodium ricotta or Cottage Cheese**: Use in moderation and choose lower-sodium varieties.

Grain and Starch Substitutions

High-Phosphorus Whole Grains

- **Substitute Brown Rice and Whole Wheat Bread** with:
  - **White Rice**: Lower in potassium and phosphorus.
  - **White Bread**: Lower in phosphorus; look for low-sodium options.
  - **Rice Cakes**: A good low-phosphorus and low-potassium snack option.

High-Potassium Cereals

- **Substitute Bran Cereals** with:
  - **Cornflakes or Rice Krispies**: Lower in potassium and phosphorus.

Vegetable Substitutions

High-Potassium Vegetables

- **Substitute Potatoes and Sweet Potatoes** with:
    - **Cauliflower**: Can be used to make a mash or rice substitute.
    - **Zucchini**: Great for roasting, grilling, or adding to salads.
- **Substitute Spinach and Swiss Chard** with:
    - **Kale**: Lower in potassium when cooked.
    - **Lettuce**: Such as romaine or iceberg, for salads and sandwiches.

Tomato Products

- **Substitute Tomato Sauce** with:
    - **Red Bell Pepper Puree**: Provides a similar texture and sweetness without the high potassium.
    - **Low-Potassium Marinara Sauce**: Make your own using peeled, deseeded tomatoes and red bell peppers.

Fruit Substitutions

High-Potassium Fruits

- **Substitute Bananas and Oranges** with:
    - **Apples**: Fresh, peeled, or as applesauce.
    - **Berries**: Blueberries, strawberries, and raspberries are great low-potassium options.

Beverage Substitutions

High-Potassium Juices

- **Substitute Orange Juice and Prune Juice** with:
    - **Apple Juice**: Lower in potassium and phosphorus.
    - **Cranberry Juice**: Good for kidney health when consumed in moderation.

High-Sodium Broths

- **Substitute Regular Chicken or Beef Broth** with:
  - **Low-Sodium Broth**: Homemade or store-bought varieties with reduced sodium content.
  - **Vegetable Broth**: Make your own with low-potassium vegetables.

Snack Substitutions

Salty Snacks

- **Substitute Potato Chips and Pretzels** with:
  - **Unsalted Popcorn**: A great low-sodium snack.
  - **Fresh Vegetables**: Carrot sticks, cucumber slices, and bell pepper strips with a CKD-friendly dip.

Sweet Treats

- **Substitute High-Sugar Desserts** with:
  - **Fresh Fruit Salad**: Use low-potassium fruits.
  - **Chia Seed Pudding**: Made with unsweetened almond milk and fresh berries.

Cooking and Seasoning Substitutions

High-Sodium Seasonings

- **Substitute Table Salt and Soy Sauce** with:
  - **Herbs and Spices**: Garlic powder, onion powder, basil, parsley, thyme, and rosemary.
  - **Salt-Free Seasoning Blends**: Such as Mrs. Dash or homemade blends.
  - **Lemon Juice or Vinegar**: For adding acidity and enhancing flavors without sodium.

High-Sodium Sauces

- **Substitute Store-Bought Salad Dressings and Marinades** with:
  - **Homemade Vinaigrettes**: Using olive oil, vinegar, and herbs.

- **Greek Yogurt-Based Dressings**: Lower in sodium and can be flavored with herbs and spices.

Tips for making healthy food choices

- Spice things up instead of using salt.
- Pile veggies like spinach, broccoli, and peppers on your pizza.
- Bake or broil your meat and fish instead of frying.
- Skip the gravy and extra fats.
- Cut back on added sugars.
- Work your way from whole milk to skim or low-fat.
- Go for whole grains like whole wheat bread, brown rice, and oats.
- Read labels to pick foods low in bad fats, salt, and sugar.
- Snack slowly—try popcorn over cake, or an orange over juice.
- Track what you eat for a week to spot when you might overdo it with high-fat or high-calorie foods.

Meal Planning

Day 1:

- **Breakfast:** Cinnamon Apple Oatmeal with Almond Milk
- **Lunch:** Grilled Chicken Breast with Roasted Vegetables and Quinoa
- **Dinner:** Baked Cod with Roasted Asparagus and Brown Rice

Day 2:

- **Breakfast:** Scrambled Eggs with Spinach and Whole Wheat Toast
- **Lunch:** Lentil Soup with Whole Wheat Bread and a Side Salad
- **Dinner:** CKD-Friendly Beef and Vegetable Stir-Fry with Brown Rice

Day 3:

- **Breakfast:** Greek Yogurt Parfait with Berries and Granola
- **Lunch:** CKD-Friendly Chicken Wrap with Lettuce, Tomato, and Avocado
- **Dinner:** Grilled Chicken Breast with Roasted Sweet Potatoes and Green Beans

Day 4:

- **Breakfast:** Avocado Toast on Whole Wheat with Poached Eggs
- **Lunch:** Tuna Salad Sandwich on Whole Wheat with Carrot Sticks
- **Dinner:** Lentil and Vegetable Curry with Brown Rice and Naan Bread

Day 5:

- **Breakfast:** CKD-Friendly Smoothie with Banana, Peanut Butter, and Almond Milk
- **Lunch:** Veggie and Bean Chili with a Side of Brown Rice
- **Dinner:** Kidney-Friendly Chicken Fajitas with Sauteed Onions and Bell Peppers

Day 6:

- **Breakfast:** Whole Grain Waffles with Fresh Strawberries and Whipped Cream
- **Lunch:** Grilled Turkey and Avocado Wrap with Mixed Greens

- **Dinner:** Roasted Chicken Thighs with Mashed Cauliflower and Steamed Broccoli

Day 7:
- **Breakfast:** High-fiber cereal with Sliced Banana and Low-Fat Milk
- **Lunch:** Kidney-Friendly Quesadilla with Shredded Chicken and Vegetables
- **Dinner:** CKD-Friendly Shrimp and Vegetable Skewers with Quinoa

Day 8:
- **Breakfast:** Veggie Omelette with Whole Wheat English Muffin
- **Lunch:** Spinach and Feta Stuffed Chicken Breast with Roasted Potatoes
- **Dinner:** Vegetable and Bean Chili with a Side of Whole Wheat Cornbread

Day 9:
- **Breakfast:** Chia Seed Pudding with Coconut Milk and Fresh Fruit
- **Lunch:** Low-Sodium Chicken Noodle Soup with Whole Wheat Crackers
- **Dinner:** Grilled Pork Chops with Roasted Brussels Sprouts and Sweet Potatoes

Day 10:
- **Breakfast:** Kidney-Friendly Breakfast Burrito with Scrambled Eggs and Black Beans
- **Lunch:** CKD-Friendly Grilled Cheese and Tomato Sandwich on Whole Wheat
- **Dinner:** CKD-Friendly Chicken and Vegetable Soup with Whole Wheat Crackers

Day 11:
- **Breakfast:** Fresh Fruit and Almond Butter Platter
- **Lunch:** CKD-Friendly Hummus with Carrot and Celery Sticks
- **Dinner:** Roasted Chickpeas Seasoned with Herbs and Spices

Day 12:
- **Breakfast:** CKD-Friendly Spinach and Artichoke Dip with Whole Wheat Pita Chips
- **Lunch:** Grilled Vegetable Skewers with Low-Fat Ranch Dip
- **Dinner:** High-fiber granola Bars with Dried Fruit and Nuts

Day 13:

- **Breakfast:** CKD-Friendly Edamame and Cherry Tomato Salad
- **Lunch:** Cucumber and Cream Cheese Roll-Ups
- **Dinner:** Fresh Fruit Salad with a Dollop of Whipped Cream

Day 14:

- **Breakfast:** CKD-Friendly Chocolate Chip Cookies with Oat Flour
- **Lunch:** Low-Sugar Banana Bread with Walnuts and Oat Flour
- **Dinner:** Kidney-Friendly No-Bake Energy Bites with Oats and Peanut Butter

Day 15:

- **Breakfast:** CKD-Friendly Vanilla Pudding with Fresh Berries and Whipped Cream
- **Lunch:** Grilled Pineapple with a Dollop of Low-Fat Yogurt
- **Dinner:** CKD-Friendly Apple Crisp with Oat Topping and Low-Fat Vanilla Ice Cream

Day 16:

- **Breakfast:** CKD-Friendly Iced Tea with Lemon and Mint
- **Lunch:** Low-Sodium Vegetable Juice with a Squeeze of Lemon
- **Dinner:** Kidney-Friendly Infused Water with Cucumber and Mint

Day 17:

- **Breakfast:** CKD-Friendly Herbal Tea with a Splash of Lemon
- **Lunch:** Low-Calorie Hot Chocolate with Almond Milk and Whipped Cream
- **Dinner:** CKD-Friendly Fresh Lemonade with a Twist of Lime

Day 18:

- **Breakfast:** Kidney-Friendly Sparkling Water with a Squeeze of Lemon
- **Lunch:** CKD-Friendly Cranberry Juice with a Splash of Water
- **Dinner:** Low-Sodium Tomato Juice with a Splash of Lemon

Day 19:

- **Breakfast:** CKD-Friendly Ginger Ale with a Squeeze of Lime
- **Lunch:** Low-Sugar Blueberry Oat Muffins
- **Dinner:** Quinoa and Black Bean Stuffed Peppers

Day 20:
- **Breakfast:** Grilled Lemon Herb Chicken with Asparagus
- **Lunch:** Zucchini Noodles with Pesto and Cherry Tomatoes
- **Dinner:** Salmon and Avocado Salad with Citrus Dressing

Day 21:
- **Breakfast:** Turkey and Vegetable Stir-Fry with Brown Rice
- **Lunch:** Cauliflower Crust Pizza with Fresh Vegetables
- **Dinner:** Chia Seed Pudding with Mixed Berries

Day 22:
- **Breakfast:** Eggplant Parmesan with Whole Wheat Pasta
- **Lunch:** Greek Yogurt Parfait with Almonds and Berries
- **Dinner:** Black Bean and Sweet Potato Tacos with Avocado

Day 23:
- **Breakfast:** Mushroom and Lentil Bolognese with Whole Wheat Pasta
- **Lunch:** Coconut Curry Lentil Soup with Naan Bread
- **Dinner:** Chickpea and Spinach Curry with Basmati Rice

Day 24:
- **Breakfast:** Cauliflower Steak with Chimichurri Sauce
- **Lunch:** Spinach and White Bean Stuffed Bell Peppers
- **Dinner:** Quinoa and Roasted Vegetable Buddha Bowl

Day 25:
- **Breakfast:** Eggplant and Chickpea Tagine with Couscous

- **Lunch:** Lentil and Vegetable Shepherd's Pie
- **Dinner:** Tofu

Day 25:

Dinner: Tofu and Vegetable Stir-Fry with Brown Rice

Day 26:

- **Breakfast:** Mushroom and Spinach Risotto with Arborio Rice
- **Lunch:** Cabbage and Carrot Slaw with Apple Cider Vinaigrette
- **Dinner:** Sesame Ginger Tofu Stir-Fry with Bok Choy

Day 27:

- **Breakfast:** Quinoa Salad with Cucumber, Tomato, and Feta
- **Lunch:** Grilled Lemon Dill Shrimp Skewers with Quinoa
- **Dinner:** Lentil and Vegetable Soup with Herbs

Day 28:

- **Breakfast:** Black Bean and Sweet Potato Tacos with Avocado
- **Lunch:** Chickpea and Spinach Curry with Basmati Rice
- **Dinner:** Eggplant and Chickpea Tagine with Couscous

Day 29:

- **Breakfast:** Mushroom and Lentil Bolognese with Whole Wheat Pasta
- **Lunch:** Cauliflower Steak with Chimichurri Sauce
- **Dinner:** Quinoa and Roasted Vegetable Buddha Bowl

Day 30:

- **Breakfast:** Spinach and White Bean Stuffed Bell Peppers
- **Lunch:** Coconut Curry Lentil Soup with Naan Bread
- **Dinner:** Tofu and Vegetable Stir-Fry with Brown Rice

Breakfast Recipes

Cinnamon Apple Oatmeal with Almond Milk

Prep Time: 5 minutes | **Cook Time:** 10 minutes | **Total Time:** 15 minutes | **Per Serving:** 2 servings

Ingredients:

- 1 cup rolled oats
- 2 cups unsweetened almond milk
- 1 medium apple, peeled, cored, and diced
- 1/2 teaspoon ground cinnamon
- 1 tablespoon honey or maple syrup (optional)
- 1/4 teaspoon vanilla extract
- Pinch of salt (optional)
- 2 tablespoons chopped walnuts (optional, for serving)

Instructions:

1. In a medium saucepan, combine the rolled oats, unsweetened almond milk, diced apple, and ground cinnamon.
2. Bring to a boil over medium heat, then reduce the heat to low and simmer for about 5-7 minutes, stirring occasionally, until the oats are cooked, and the mixture is creamy.
3. Stir in the honey or maple syrup (if using) and vanilla extract.
4. Remove from heat and let it sit for a minute.
5. Serve warm, topped with chopped walnuts if desired.

Nutritional Value: Calories: 250 | Phosphorus: 120 mg | Sodium: 60 mg | Protein: 5 g | Carbohydrates: 40 g | Fats: 7 g | Potassium: 200 mg | Iron: 2 mg

Scrambled Eggs with Spinach and Whole Wheat Toast

Prep Time: 5 minutes | **Cook Time:** 5 minutes | **Total Time:** 10 minutes | **Per Serving:** 2 servings

Ingredients:

- 4 large eggs
- 1 cup fresh spinach, chopped
- 1/4 cup unsweetened almond milk
- 1 tablespoon olive oil
- Salt and pepper, to taste
- 2 slices whole wheat toast

Instructions:

1. In a bowl, whisk together the eggs, unsweetened almond milk, salt, and pepper.
2. Heat the olive oil in a non-stick skillet over medium heat.
3. Add the chopped spinach to the skillet and cook until wilted, about 1-2 minutes.
4. Pour the egg mixture into the skillet and cook, stirring gently, until the eggs are set, about 3-4 minutes.
5. Serve the scrambled eggs with spinach alongside whole wheat toast.

Nutritional Value: Calories: 220 | Phosphorus: 190 mg | Sodium: 150 mg | Protein: 12 g | Carbohydrates: 20 g | Fats: 10 g | Potassium: 250 mg | Iron: 3 mg

Greek Yogurt Parfait with Berries and Granola

Prep Time: 5 minutes | **Cook Time:** 0 minutes | **Total Time:** 5 minutes | **Per Serving:** 2 servings

Ingredients:

- 1 cup Greek yogurt (low phosphorus and potassium variety)
- 1/2 cup mixed berries (strawberries, blueberries, raspberries)
- 1/4 cup low-sugar granola
- 1 tablespoon honey (optional)

Instructions:

1. In a glass or bowl, layer half of the Greek yogurt, followed by half of the mixed berries, and half of the granola.
2. Repeat the layers with the remaining Greek yogurt, berries, and granola.
3. Drizzle with honey if desired.
4. Serve immediately.

Nutritional Value: Calories: 200 | Phosphorus: 150 mg | Sodium: 60 mg | Protein: 10 g | Carbohydrates: 25 g | Fats: 5 g | Potassium: 200 mg | Iron: 1 mg

Avocado Toast on Whole Wheat with Poached Eggs

Prep Time: 10 minutes | **Cook Time:** 5 minutes | **Total Time:** 15 minutes | **Per Serving:** 2 servings

Ingredients:

- 2 slices whole wheat bread
- 1 ripe avocado, mashed
- 2 large eggs
- 1 tablespoon white vinegar
- Salt and pepper, to taste
- Red pepper flakes (optional)

Instructions:

1. Toast the whole wheat bread slices until golden brown.
2. Spread the mashed avocado evenly on each toast.
3. Bring a medium pot of water to a gentle simmer and add the white vinegar.
4. Crack each egg into a small bowl and gently slide them into the simmering water.
5. Poach the eggs for about 3-4 minutes, until the whites are set but the yolks are still runny.
6. Using a slotted spoon, carefully remove the eggs from the water and place one on each avocado toast.
7. Season with salt, pepper, and red pepper flakes if desired.
8. Serve immediately.

Nutritional Value: Calories: 300 | Phosphorus: 220 mg | Sodium: 170 mg | Protein: 10 g | Carbohydrates: 30 g | Fats: 15 g | Potassium: 400 mg | Iron: 2 mg

CKD-Friendly Smoothie with Banana, Peanut Butter, and Almond Milk

Prep Time: 5 minutes | **Cook Time:** 0 minutes | **Total Time:** 5 minutes | **Per Serving:** 2 servings

Ingredients:

- 1 medium banana
- 2 tablespoons peanut butter (unsalted)
- 1 cup unsweetened almond milk
- 1/2 cup ice cubes
- 1 teaspoon honey (optional)

Instructions:

1. In a blender, combine the banana, peanut butter, unsweetened almond milk, and ice cubes.
2. Blend until smooth and creamy.
3. Add honey if desired and blend again.
4. Pour into glasses and serve immediately.

Nutritional Value: Calories: 250 | Phosphorus: 120 mg | Sodium: 70 mg | Protein: 6 g | Carbohydrates: 30 g | Fats: 12 g | Potassium: 300 mg | Iron: 1 mg

Whole Grain Waffles with Fresh Strawberries and Whipped Cream

Prep Time: 10 minutes | **Cook Time:** 15 minutes | **Total Time:** 25 minutes | **Per Serving:** 4 servings

Ingredients:

- 1 1/2 cups whole grain waffle mix
- 1 cup water
- 1 tablespoon olive oil
- 1 cup fresh strawberries, sliced
- 1/2 cup whipped cream (low-fat)

Instructions:

1. Preheat your waffle iron according to the manufacturer's instructions.
2. In a large bowl, combine the whole-grain waffle mix, water, and olive oil. Stir until just combined.
3. Pour the batter onto the preheated waffle iron and cook until golden brown and crisp.
4. Top the waffles with fresh strawberries and a dollop of whipped cream.
5. Serve immediately.

Nutritional Value: Calories: 250 | Phosphorus: 150 mg | Sodium: 200 mg | Protein: 6 g | Carbohydrates: 40 g | Fats: 8 g | Potassium: 150 mg | Iron: 2 mg

High-fiber cereal with Sliced Banana and Low-Fat Milk

Prep Time: 5 minutes | **Cook Time:** 0 minutes | **Total Time:** 5 minutes | **Per Serving:** 2 servings

Ingredients:

- 2 cups high-fiber cereal (low-sodium)
- 1 medium banana, sliced
- 2 cups low-fat milk (or unsweetened almond milk)

Instructions:

1. Divide the cereal evenly between two bowls.
2. Top each bowl with sliced banana.
3. Pour 1 cup of low-fat milk over each bowl of cereal.
4. Serve immediately.

Nutritional Value: Calories: 300 | Phosphorus: 200 mg | Sodium: 150 mg | Protein: 8 g | Carbohydrates: 60 g | Fats: 4 g | Potassium: 400 mg | Iron: 3 mg

Veggie Omelette with Whole Wheat English Muffin

Prep Time: 10 minutes | **Cook Time:** 10 minutes | **Total Time:** 20 minutes | **Per Serving:** 2 servings

Ingredients:

- 4 large eggs
- 1/2 cup chopped bell peppers
- 1/2 cup chopped onions
- 1/2 cup chopped mushrooms
- 1 tablespoon olive oil
- Salt and pepper, to taste
- 2 whole wheat English muffins, toasted

Instructions:

1. In a bowl, whisk together the eggs, salt, and pepper.
2. Heat olive oil in a non-stick skillet over medium heat.
3. Add the chopped bell peppers, onions, and mushrooms to the skillet and sauté until softened, about 3-4 minutes.
4. Pour the egg mixture over the vegetables and cook, lifting the edges occasionally to let uncooked egg flow underneath, until the omelet is set about 5 minutes.
5. Fold the omelet in half and transfer to a plate.
6. Serve the omelet with toasted whole wheat English muffins.

Nutritional Value: Calories: 350 | Phosphorus: 250 mg | Sodium: 220 mg | Protein: 18 g | Carbohydrates: 30 g | Fats: 18 g | Potassium: 350 mg | Iron: 3 mg

Chia Seed Pudding with Coconut Milk and Fresh Fruit

Prep Time: 5 minutes | **Cook Time:** 0 minutes | **Total Time:** 5 minutes (plus chilling time) | **Per Serving:** 2 servings

Ingredients:

- 1/4 cup chia seeds
- 1 cup unsweetened coconut milk
- 1 tablespoon honey (optional)
- 1/2 teaspoon vanilla extract
- 1/2 cup fresh fruit (berries, apple slices, or pear slices)

Instructions:

1. In a bowl, combine chia seeds, coconut milk, honey (if using), and vanilla extract. Stir well to combine.
2. Cover and refrigerate for at least 2 hours or overnight, until the mixture has thickened to a pudding-like consistency.
3. Stir the pudding before serving.
4. Top with fresh fruit.
5. Serve chilled.

Nutritional Value: Calories: 200 | Phosphorus: 120 mg | Sodium: 30 mg | Protein: 4 g | Carbohydrates: 25 g | Fats: 10 g | Potassium: 200 mg | Iron: 2 mg

Kidney-Friendly Breakfast Burrito with Scrambled Eggs and Black Beans

Prep Time: 10 minutes | **Cook Time:** 10 minutes | **Total Time:** 20 minutes | **Per Serving:** 2 servings

Ingredients:

- 4 large eggs
- 1/4 cup unsweetened almond milk
- 1/2 cup canned black beans, drained, and rinsed
- 1/2 cup chopped bell peppers
- 1/4 cup chopped onions
- 1 tablespoon olive oil
- 2 whole wheat tortillas
- Salt and pepper, to taste
- 1/4 cup salsa (low sodium, optional)

Instructions:

1. In a bowl, whisk together the eggs, almond milk, salt, and pepper.
2. Heat olive oil in a non-stick skillet over medium heat.
3. Add the chopped bell peppers and onions to the skillet and sauté until softened, about 3-4 minutes.
4. Add the black beans and cook until heated through about 2 minutes.
5. Pour the egg mixture into the skillet and cook, stirring gently, until the eggs are scrambled and cooked through.
6. Warm the tortillas in a separate skillet or microwave.
7. Divide the scrambled egg mixture between the two tortillas.
8. Add salsa if desired.
9. Roll up the tortillas to form burritos.
10. Serve immediately.

Nutritional Value: Calories: 300 | Phosphorus: 220 mg | Sodium: 180 mg | Protein: 15 g | Carbohydrates: 35 g | Fats: 10 g | Potassium: 350 mg | Iron: 3 mg

Lunch Recipes

Grilled Chicken Breast with Roasted Vegetables and Quinoa

Prep Time: 10 minutes | **Cook Time:** 30 minutes | **Total Time:** 40 minutes | **Per Serving:** 4 servings

Ingredients:

- 4 boneless, skinless chicken breasts
- 2 tablespoons olive oil
- 1 teaspoon dried thyme
- 1 teaspoon dried rosemary
- 1 teaspoon garlic powder
- Salt and pepper, to taste
- 2 cups mixed vegetables (zucchini, bell peppers, and onions), chopped
- 1 cup quinoa
- 2 cups water
- 1 tablespoon lemon juice

Instructions:

1. Preheat the grill to medium-high heat.
2. Brush the chicken breasts with 1 tablespoon of olive oil and season with dried thyme, rosemary, garlic powder, salt, and pepper.
3. Grill the chicken for 6-7 minutes on each side, or until fully cooked.
4. Preheat the oven to 400°F (200°C). Toss the mixed vegetables with the remaining olive oil, salt, and pepper, then spread them on a baking sheet.
5. Roast the vegetables in the oven for 20-25 minutes, until tender.
6. Meanwhile, rinse the quinoa under cold water. In a medium saucepan, bring the quinoa and water to a boil. Reduce to a simmer, cover, and cook for 15 minutes or until the quinoa is tender and the water is absorbed.
7. Fluff the quinoa with a fork and stir in the lemon juice.
8. Serve the grilled chicken with roasted vegetables and quinoa.

Nutritional Value: Calories: 350 | Phosphorus: 250 mg | Sodium: 100 mg | Protein: 30 g | Carbohydrates: 30 g | Fats: 12 g | Potassium: 400 mg | Iron: 4 mg

Lentil Soup with Whole Wheat Bread and a Side Salad

Prep Time: 10 minutes | **Cook Time:** 30 minutes | **Total Time:** 40 minutes | **Per Serving:** 4 servings

Ingredients:

- 1 cup dried lentils, rinsed
- 1 tablespoon olive oil
- 1 onion, chopped
- 2 carrots, chopped
- 2 celery stalks, chopped
- 3 cloves garlic, minced
- 6 cups low-sodium vegetable broth
- 1 teaspoon dried thyme
- 1 bay leaf
- Salt and pepper, to taste
- 4 slices whole wheat bread
- 4 cups mixed salad greens
- 1 cucumber, sliced
- 1/2 cup cherry tomatoes, halved
- 1 tablespoon balsamic vinegar

Instructions:

1. In a large pot, heat the olive oil over medium heat. Add the onion, carrots, celery, and garlic. Cook until the vegetables are softened, about 5 minutes.
2. Add the lentils, vegetable broth, dried thyme, bay leaf, salt, and pepper. Bring to a boil, then reduce the heat and simmer for 25-30 minutes, until the lentils are tender.
3. Remove the bay leaf before serving.
4. Toast the whole wheat bread slices.
5. In a large bowl, combine the mixed salad greens, cucumber, and cherry tomatoes. Drizzle with balsamic vinegar.
6. Serve the lentil soup with toasted whole wheat bread and a side salad.

Nutritional Value: Calories: 300 | Phosphorus: 220 mg | Sodium: 150 mg | Protein: 12 g | Carbohydrates: 50 g | Fats: 6 g | Potassium: 500 mg | Iron: 5 mg

CKD-Friendly Chicken Wrap with Lettuce, Tomato, and Avocado

Prep Time: 10 minutes | **Cook Time:** 10 minutes | **Total Time:** 20 minutes | **Per Serving:** 2 servings

Ingredients:

- 2 boneless, skinless chicken breasts
- 1 tablespoon olive oil
- 1/2 teaspoon garlic powder
- 1/2 teaspoon paprika
- Salt and pepper, to taste
- 2 whole wheat tortillas
- 1 cup lettuce, shredded
- 1 tomato, sliced
- 1/2 avocado, sliced

Instructions:

1. Heat the olive oil in a skillet over medium heat. Season the chicken breasts with garlic powder, paprika, salt, and pepper.
2. Cook the chicken in the skillet for 5-7 minutes on each side, until fully cooked. Remove from heat and let it rest for a few minutes before slicing thinly.
3. Warm the whole wheat tortillas in a skillet or microwave.
4. Place the sliced chicken, lettuce, tomato, and avocado on each tortilla.
5. Roll up the tortillas to form wraps.
6. Serve immediately.

Nutritional Value: Calories: 350 | Phosphorus: 200 mg | Sodium: 150 mg | Protein: 28 g | Carbohydrates: 30 g | Fats: 14 g | Potassium: 450 mg | Iron: 2 mg

Tuna Salad Sandwich on Whole Wheat with Carrot Sticks

Prep Time: 10 minutes | **Cook Time:** 0 minutes | **Total Time:** 10 minutes | **Per Serving:** 2 servings

Ingredients:

- 1 can (5 ounces) tuna packed in water, drained
- 2 tablespoons plain Greek yogurt
- 1 teaspoon Dijon mustard
- 1 celery stalk, finely chopped
- 1 tablespoon red onion, finely chopped
- 4 slices whole wheat bread
- Lettuce leaves
- 2 medium carrots, cut into sticks

Instructions:

1. In a bowl, combine the drained tuna, Greek yogurt, Dijon mustard, celery, and red onion. Mix well.
2. Spread the tuna salad evenly on two slices of whole wheat bread. Top with lettuce leaves and the remaining bread slices.
3. Serve with carrot sticks on the side.

Nutritional Value: Calories: 300 | Phosphorus: 150 mg | Sodium: 200 mg | Protein: 20 g | Carbohydrates: 35 g | Fats: 8 g | Potassium: 400 mg | Iron: 3 mg

Veggie and Bean Chili with a Side of Brown Rice

Prep Time: 15 minutes | **Cook Time:** 30 minutes | **Total Time:** 45 minutes | **Per Serving:** 4 servings

Ingredients:

- 1 tablespoon olive oil
- 1 onion, chopped
- 2 cloves garlic, minced
- 1 bell pepper, chopped
- 1 zucchini, chopped
- 1 cup canned kidney beans, drained and rinsed
- 1 cup canned black beans, drained, and rinsed
- 2 cups low-sodium vegetable broth
- 1 can (14.5 ounces) diced tomatoes; no salt added
- 1 tablespoon chili powder
- 1 teaspoon ground cumin
- 1 teaspoon smoked paprika
- Salt and pepper, to taste
- 1 cup brown rice
- 2 cups water

Instructions:

1. In a large pot, heat the olive oil over medium heat. Add the onion and garlic and cook until softened about 3 minutes.
2. Add the bell pepper and zucchini and cook for another 5 minutes.
3. Stir in the kidney beans, black beans, vegetable broth, diced tomatoes, chili powder, cumin, smoked paprika, salt, and pepper. Bring to a boil, then reduce the heat and simmer for 20-25 minutes.
4. While the chili is simmering, rinse the brown rice under cold water. In a medium saucepan, bring the rice and water to a boil. Reduce to a simmer, cover, and cook for 20 minutes or until the rice is tender and the water is absorbed.
5. Serve the veggie and bean chili over brown rice.

Nutritional Value: Calories: 400 | Phosphorus: 250 mg | Sodium: 150 mg | Protein: 15 g | Carbohydrates: 70 g | Fats: 8 g | Potassium: 600 mg | Iron: 6 mg

Grilled Turkey and Avocado Wrap with Mixed Greens

Prep Time: 10 minutes | **Cook Time:** 0 minutes | **Total Time:** 10 minutes | **Per Serving:** 2 servings

Ingredients:

- 4 slices of low-sodium turkey breast
- 1/2 avocado, sliced
- 2 cups mixed greens
- 1 small tomato, sliced
- 2 whole wheat tortillas
- 1 tablespoon olive oil
- 1 tablespoon lemon juice
- Salt and pepper, to taste

Instructions:

1. In a small bowl, whisk together the olive oil, lemon juice, salt, and pepper.
2. Lay the whole wheat tortillas flat and arrange 2 slices of turkey breast on each.
3. Top with avocado slices, mixed greens, and tomato slices.
4. Drizzle with the olive oil and lemon juice mixture.
5. Roll up the tortillas to form wraps.
6. Serve immediately.

Nutritional Value: Calories: 320 | Phosphorus: 200 mg | Sodium: 250 mg | Protein: 20 g | Carbohydrates: 30 g | Fats: 15 g | Potassium: 400 mg | Iron: 2 mg

Kidney-friendly quesadilla with Shredded Chicken and Vegetables

Prep Time: 10 minutes | **Cook Time:** 10 minutes | **Total Time:** 20 minutes | **Per Serving:** 2 servings

Ingredients:

- 1 cup cooked, shredded chicken breast
- 1/2 cup bell peppers, chopped
- 1/2 cup onions, chopped
- 1 cup low-fat shredded cheese (low sodium)
- 2 whole wheat tortillas
- 1 tablespoon olive oil
- 1 teaspoon cumin
- Salt and pepper, to taste

Instructions:

1. Heat the olive oil in a skillet over medium heat. Add the bell peppers and onions, and sauté until softened, about 5 minutes.
2. Add the shredded chicken, cumin, salt, and pepper. Stir to combine and cook until heated through.
3. Place a tortilla in a separate skillet over medium heat. Sprinkle half of the cheese on one half of the tortilla, then add half of the chicken and vegetable mixture.
4. Fold the tortilla over and cook until the cheese is melted, and the tortilla is golden brown, about 2-3 minutes per side.
5. Repeat with the second tortilla and remaining ingredients.
6. Cut each quesadilla into wedges and serve immediately.

Nutritional Value: Calories: 350 | Phosphorus: 230 mg | Sodium: 250 mg | Protein: 25 g | Carbohydrates: 30 g | Fats: 15 g | Potassium: 350 mg | Iron: 2 mg

Spinach and Feta Stuffed Chicken Breast with Roasted Potatoes

Prep Time: 15 minutes | **Cook Time:** 30 minutes | **Total Time:** 45 minutes | **Per Serving:** 4 servings

Ingredients:

- 4 boneless, skinless chicken breasts
- 1 cup fresh spinach, chopped
- 1/2 cup crumbled feta cheese (low sodium)
- 1 tablespoon olive oil
- 1 teaspoon dried oregano
- Salt and pepper, to taste
- 4 medium potatoes, cut into wedges
- 1 tablespoon olive oil
- 1 teaspoon rosemary, chopped

Instructions:

1. Preheat the oven to 400°F (200°C).
2. In a small bowl, mix the chopped spinach and feta cheese.
3. Cut a horizontal slit in each chicken breast to form a pocket. Stuff each pocket with the spinach and feta mixture.
4. Secure the openings with toothpicks if necessary. Season the chicken breasts with dried oregano, salt, and pepper.
5. Heat the olive oil in a large oven-safe skillet over medium heat. Sear the chicken breasts until golden brown on each side, about 3-4 minutes per side.
6. Transfer the skillet to the oven and bake for 20 minutes, or until the chicken is fully cooked.
7. While the chicken is baking, toss the potato wedges with olive oil, rosemary, salt, and pepper. Spread them on a baking sheet and roast in the oven for 25-30 minutes, until golden and crispy.
8. Serve the stuffed chicken breasts with roasted potatoes.

Nutritional Value: Calories: 400 | Phosphorus: 250 mg | Sodium: 280 mg | Protein: 30 g | Carbohydrates: 35 g | Fats: 15 g | Potassium: 500 mg | Iron: 3 mg

Low-sodium chicken Noodle Soup with Whole Wheat Crackers

Prep Time: 15 minutes | **Cook Time:** 30 minutes | **Total Time:** 45 minutes | **Per Serving:** 4 servings

Ingredients:

- 1 tablespoon olive oil
- 1 onion, chopped
- 2 carrots, chopped
- 2 celery stalks, chopped
- 2 cloves garlic, minced
- 6 cups low-sodium chicken broth
- 1 cup cooked chicken breast, shredded
- 1 cup whole wheat noodles
- 1 teaspoon dried thyme
- 1 bay leaf
- Salt and pepper, to taste
- 16 whole wheat crackers

Instructions:

1. In a large pot, heat the olive oil over medium heat. Add the onion, carrots, and celery. Cook until the vegetables are softened, about 5 minutes.
2. Add the garlic and cook for another minute.
3. Pour in the low-sodium chicken broth and bring to a boil.
4. Add the shredded chicken, whole wheat noodles, dried thyme, bay leaf, salt, and pepper. Reduce the heat and simmer for 20 minutes, or until the noodles are tender.
5. Remove the bay leaf before serving.
6. Serve the soup with whole wheat crackers on the side.

Nutritional Value: Calories: 300 | Phosphorus: 150 mg | Sodium: 150 mg | Protein: 20 g | Carbohydrates: 40 g | Fats: 8 g | Potassium: 400 mg | Iron: 2 mg

CKD-Friendly Grilled Cheese and Tomato Sandwich on Whole Wheat

Prep Time: 5 minutes | **Cook Time:** 10 minutes | **Total Time:** 15 minutes | **Per Serving:** 2 servings

Ingredients:

- 4 slices whole wheat bread
- 4 slices low-sodium cheese
- 1 tomato, sliced
- 2 tablespoons unsalted butter

Instructions:

1. Heat a skillet over medium heat.
2. Butter one side of each slice of whole wheat bread.
3. Place two slices of bread, butter side down, in the skillet.
4. Top each with 2 slices of low-sodium cheese and tomato slices.
5. Place the remaining slices of bread on top, butter side up.
6. Cook until the bread is golden brown, and the cheese is melted, about 3-4 minutes per side.
7. Serve immediately.

Nutritional Value: Calories: 350 | Phosphorus: 180 mg | Sodium: 200 mg | Protein: 15 g | Carbohydrates: 35 g | Fats: 18 g | Potassium: 350 mg | Iron: 2 mg

Dinner Recipes

Baked Cod with Roasted Asparagus and Brown Rice

Prep Time: 10 minutes | **Cook Time:** 25 minutes | **Total Time:** 35 minutes | **Per Serving:** 4 servings

Ingredients:

- 4 cod fillets
- 1 tablespoon olive oil
- 1 teaspoon dried thyme
- 1 lemon, sliced
- Salt and pepper, to taste
- 1 bunch asparagus, trimmed
- 1 cup brown rice
- 2 cups water

Instructions:

1. Preheat the oven to 400°F (200°C).
2. Rinse the brown rice under cold water and combine with 2 cups of water in a medium pot. Bring to a boil, reduce heat to low, cover, and simmer for 25 minutes or until the rice is tender.
3. Place the cod fillets on a baking sheet lined with parchment paper. Drizzle with olive oil and sprinkle with dried thyme, salt, and pepper. Top each fillet with lemon slices.
4. Arrange the asparagus next to the cod fillets on the baking sheet. Drizzle with a little olive oil, and season with salt and pepper.
5. Bake for 20 minutes, or until the cod is cooked through and the asparagus is tender.
6. Serve the baked cod with roasted asparagus and brown rice.

Nutritional Value: Calories: 350 | Phosphorus: 220 mg | Sodium: 180 mg | Protein: 25 g | Carbohydrates: 45 g | Fats: 10 g | Potassium: 450 mg | Iron: 3 mg

CKD-Friendly Beef and Vegetable Stir-Fry with Brown Rice

Prep Time: 10 minutes | **Cook Time:** 15 minutes | **Total Time:** 25 minutes | **Per Serving:** 4 servings

Ingredients:

- 1-pound lean beef sirloin, thinly sliced
- 2 tablespoons olive oil
- 1 bell pepper, sliced
- 1 cup broccoli florets
- 1 cup snap peas
- 2 cloves garlic, minced
- 1 tablespoon low-sodium soy sauce
- 1 tablespoon rice vinegar
- 1 teaspoon ground ginger
- 1 cup brown rice
- 2 cups water

Instructions:

1. Rinse the brown rice under cold water and combine with 2 cups of water in a medium pot. Bring to a boil, reduce heat to low, cover, and simmer for 25 minutes or until the rice is tender.
2. In a large skillet, heat 1 tablespoon of olive oil over medium-high heat. Add the beef slices and cook until browned about 5 minutes. Remove the beef from the skillet and set aside.
3. Add the remaining olive oil to the skillet and sauté the bell pepper, broccoli, snap peas, and garlic for about 5 minutes, or until tender-crisp.
4. Return the beef to the skillet and add the low-sodium soy sauce, rice vinegar, and ground ginger. Stir to combine and cook for another 2-3 minutes, until heated through.
5. Serve the beef and vegetable stir-fry over brown rice.

Nutritional Value: Calories: 400 | Phosphorus: 230 mg | Sodium: 200 mg | Protein: 30 g | Carbohydrates: 40 g | Fats: 15 g | Potassium: 450 mg | Iron: 4 mg

Grilled Chicken Breast with Roasted Sweet Potatoes and Green Beans

Prep Time: 10 minutes | **Cook Time:** 25 minutes | **Total Time:** 35 minutes | **Per Serving:** 4 servings

Ingredients:

- 4 chicken breasts
- 2 tablespoons olive oil
- 1 teaspoon paprika
- Salt and pepper, to taste
- 2 large, sweet potatoes, peeled and cut into wedges
- 1-pound green beans, trimmed
- 1 tablespoon fresh lemon juice

Instructions:

1. Preheat the oven to 400°F (200°C).
2. In a large bowl, toss the sweet potato wedges with 1 tablespoon of olive oil, paprika, salt, and pepper. Spread them out on a baking sheet.
3. Place the green beans on a separate baking sheet and toss with the remaining olive oil, salt, and pepper.
4. Bake the sweet potatoes and green beans for 20-25 minutes, until tender and golden brown.
5. Meanwhile, heat a grill pan over medium-high heat. Season the chicken breasts with salt, pepper, and lemon juice. Grill the chicken for 5-7 minutes on each side, or until fully cooked.
6. Serve the grilled chicken breasts with roasted sweet potatoes and green beans.

Nutritional Value: Calories: 400 | Phosphorus: 250 mg | Sodium: 180 mg | Protein: 35 g | Carbohydrates: 45 g | Fats: 10 g | Potassium: 600 mg | Iron: 3 mg

Lentil and Vegetable Curry with Brown Rice and Naan Bread

Prep Time: 15 minutes | **Cook Time:** 30 minutes | **Total Time:** 45 minutes | **Per Serving:** 4 servings

Ingredients:

- 1 cup dried lentils, rinsed
- 2 tablespoons olive oil
- 1 onion, chopped
- 2 cloves garlic, minced
- 1 tablespoon curry powder
- 1 teaspoon ground cumin
- 1 teaspoon ground turmeric
- 1 cup diced tomatoes (no salt added)
- 2 cups low-sodium vegetable broth
- 1 cup cauliflower florets
- 1 cup carrots, chopped
- 1 cup spinach leaves
- 1 cup brown rice
- 2 cups water
- 4 small pieces of naan bread (low sodium if possible)

Instructions:

1. Rinse the brown rice under cold water and combine with 2 cups of water in a medium pot. Bring to a boil, reduce heat to low, cover, and simmer for 25 minutes or until the rice is tender.
2. In a large pot, heat the olive oil over medium heat. Add the onion and garlic, and sauté until the onion is translucent, about 5 minutes.
3. Stir in the curry powder, cumin, and turmeric, and cook for another minute.
4. Add the lentils, diced tomatoes, and vegetable broth. Bring to a boil, then reduce the heat and simmer for 20 minutes.
5. Add the cauliflower and carrots and continue to cook until the vegetables are tender about 10 minutes.
6. Stir in the spinach leaves and cook until wilted about 2 minutes.
7. Serve the lentil and vegetable curry over brown rice with a side of naan bread.

Nutritional Value: Calories: 450 | Phosphorus: 300 mg | Sodium: 200 mg | Protein: 20 g | Carbohydrates: 70 g | Fats: 10 g | Potassium: 600 mg | Iron: 5 mg

Kidney-Friendly Chicken Fajitas with Sauteed Onions and Bell Peppers

Prep Time: 10 minutes | **Cook Time:** 15 minutes | **Total Time:** 25 minutes | **Per Serving:** 4 servings

Ingredients:

- 1 pound chicken breast, thinly sliced
- 2 tablespoons olive oil
- 1 onion, sliced
- 2 bell peppers, sliced
- 1 teaspoon ground cumin
- 1 teaspoon paprika
- Salt and pepper, to taste
- 8 small whole wheat tortillas
- 1 lime, cut into wedges
- Fresh cilantro, chopped (optional)

Instructions:

1. Heat 1 tablespoon of olive oil in a large skillet over medium-high heat. Add the chicken slices and cook until browned and cooked through about 5-7 minutes. Remove the chicken from the skillet and set aside.
2. Add the remaining olive oil to the skillet and sauté the onions and bell peppers until tender, about 5 minutes.
3. Return the chicken to the skillet and season with ground cumin, paprika, salt, and pepper. Stir to combine and cook for another 2-3 minutes.
4. Warm the whole wheat tortillas in a separate pan or microwave.
5. Serve the chicken fajitas with lime wedges and chopped cilantro, if desired.

Nutritional Value: Calories: 350 | Phosphorus: 200 mg | Sodium: 180 mg | Protein: 25 g | Carbohydrates: 40 g | Fats: 10 g | Potassium: 450 mg | Iron: 3 mg

Roasted Chicken Thighs with Mashed Cauliflower and Steamed Broccoli

Prep Time: 10 minutes | **Cook Time:** 35 minutes | **Total Time:** 45 minutes | **Per Serving:** 4 servings

Ingredients:

- 4 bone-in, skinless chicken thighs
- 2 tablespoons olive oil
- 1 teaspoon dried thyme
- Salt and pepper, to taste
- 1 head cauliflower, chopped
- 1/4 cup unsweetened almond milk
- 1 tablespoon unsalted butter
- 1 pound broccoli florets, steamed

Instructions:

1. Preheat the oven to 400°F (200°C).
2. Rub the chicken thighs with olive oil, thyme, salt, and pepper. Place them on a baking sheet lined with parchment paper.
3. Roast the chicken thighs for 30-35 minutes, or until the internal temperature reaches 165°F (75°C).
4. Meanwhile, steam the cauliflower until tender, about 10 minutes. Drain and transfer to a food processor.
5. Add the almond milk and butter to the cauliflower, and blend until smooth. Season with salt and pepper to taste.
6. Steam the broccoli florets until tender, about 5-7 minutes.
7. Serve the roasted chicken thighs with mashed cauliflower and steamed broccoli.

Nutritional Value: Calories: 350 | Phosphorus: 200 mg | Sodium: 180 mg | Protein: 25 g | Carbohydrates: 20 g | Fats: 20 g | Potassium: 400 mg | Iron: 2 mg

CKD-Friendly Shrimp and Vegetable Skewers with Quinoa

Prep Time: 15 minutes | **Cook Time:** 20 minutes | **Total Time:** 35 minutes | **Per Serving:** 4 servings

Ingredients:

- 1-pound large shrimp, peeled and deveined
- 1 red bell pepper, cut into chunks
- 1 yellow bell pepper, cut into chunks
- 1 zucchini, sliced
- 2 tablespoons olive oil
- 1 teaspoon dried oregano
- Salt and pepper, to taste
- 1 cup quinoa
- 2 cups water

Instructions:

1. Rinse the quinoa under cold water and combine with 2 cups of water in a medium pot. Bring to a boil, reduce heat to low, cover, and simmer for 15 minutes or until the quinoa is tender.
2. Preheat the grill to medium-high heat.
3. Thread the shrimp, bell peppers, and zucchini onto skewers. Brush with olive oil and sprinkle with oregano, salt, and pepper.
4. Grill the skewers for 3-4 minutes on each side, until the shrimp are opaque, and the vegetables are tender.
5. Serve the shrimp and vegetable skewers over cooked quinoa.

Nutritional Value: Calories: 350 | Phosphorus: 250 mg | Sodium: 190 mg | Protein: 25 g | Carbohydrates: 30 g | Fats: 15 g | Potassium: 450 mg | Iron: 3 mg

Vegetable and Bean Chili with a Side of Whole Wheat Cornbread

Prep Time: 15 minutes | **Cook Time:** 30 minutes | **Total Time:** 45 minutes | **Per Serving:** 4 servings

Ingredients:

- 1 tablespoon olive oil
- 1 onion, chopped
- 2 cloves garlic, minced
- 1 bell pepper, chopped
- 1 zucchini, chopped
- 1 can (15 ounces) low-sodium black beans, rinsed and drained
- 1 can (15 ounces) no-salt-added diced tomatoes
- 1 cup low-sodium vegetable broth
- 1 tablespoon chili powder
- 1 teaspoon cumin
- 1 teaspoon paprika
- Salt and pepper, to taste
- 1 cup whole wheat cornmeal
- 1 cup low-fat buttermilk
- 1 egg
- 1 tablespoon honey

Instructions:

1. Preheat the oven to 400°F (200°C).
2. In a large pot, heat the olive oil over medium heat. Add the onion and garlic, and sauté until the onion is translucent, about 5 minutes.
3. Add the bell pepper and zucchini and cook for another 5 minutes.
4. Stir in the black beans, diced tomatoes, vegetable broth, chili powder, cumin, and paprika. Bring to a boil, then reduce the heat and simmer for 20 minutes.
5. Meanwhile, in a bowl, mix the cornmeal, buttermilk, egg, and honey. Pour into a greased baking dish and bake for 15-20 minutes, until golden brown.
6. Serve the vegetable and bean chili with a side of whole wheat cornbread.

Nutritional Value: Calories: 400 | Phosphorus: 200 mg | Sodium: 150 mg | Protein: 12 g | Carbohydrates: 60 g | Fats: 10 g | Potassium: 500 mg | Iron: 3 mg

Grilled Pork Chops with Roasted Brussels Sprouts and Sweet Potatoes

Prep Time: 10 minutes | **Cook Time:** 30 minutes | **Total Time:** 40 minutes | **Per Serving:** 4 servings

Ingredients:

- 4 boneless pork chops
- 2 tablespoons olive oil
- 1 teaspoon dried rosemary
- Salt and pepper, to taste
- 1 pound Brussels sprouts, halved
- 2 large, sweet potatoes, peeled and cubed
- 1 tablespoon balsamic vinegar

Instructions:

1. Preheat the oven to 400°F (200°C).
2. In a large bowl, toss the Brussels sprouts and sweet potatoes with 1 tablespoon of olive oil, salt, and pepper. Spread them out on a baking sheet.
3. Roast the vegetables for 25-30 minutes, until tender and golden brown.
4. Meanwhile, heat a grill pan over medium-high heat. Rub the pork chops with the remaining olive oil, rosemary, salt, and pepper.
5. Grill the pork chops for 4-5 minutes on each side, until cooked through.
6. Drizzle the roasted vegetables with balsamic vinegar and serve alongside the grilled pork chops.

Nutritional Value: Calories: 450 | Phosphorus: 250 mg | Sodium: 180 mg | Protein: 30 g | Carbohydrates: 45 g | Fats: 20 g | Potassium: 600 mg | Iron: 3 mg

CKD-Friendly Chicken and Vegetable Soup with Whole Wheat Crackers

Prep Time: 10 minutes | **Cook Time:** 20 minutes | **Total Time:** 30 minutes | **Per Serving:** 4 servings

Ingredients:

- 1 tablespoon olive oil
- 1 onion, chopped
- 2 cloves garlic, minced
- 2 carrots, sliced
- 2 celery stalks, sliced
- 1 zucchini, chopped
- 1 cup low-sodium chicken broth
- 2 cups water
- 1 cup cooked chicken breast, shredded
- 1 teaspoon dried thyme
- Salt and pepper, to taste
- 1 cup whole wheat crackers

Instructions:

1. In a large pot, heat the olive oil over medium heat. Add the onion and garlic, and sauté until the onion is translucent, about 5 minutes.
2. Add the carrots, celery, and zucchini, and cook for another 5 minutes.
3. Pour in the chicken broth and water and bring to a boil. Reduce the heat and simmer for 10 minutes.
4. Stir in the shredded chicken and thyme. Season with salt and pepper to taste.
5. Serve the soup with whole wheat crackers on the side.

Nutritional Value: Calories: 300 | Phosphorus: 150 mg | Sodium: 140 mg | Protein: 20 g | Carbohydrates: 30 g | Fats: 10 g | Potassium: 450 mg | Iron: 2 mg

Snacks and Appetizers

Fresh Fruit and Almond Butter Platter

Prep Time: 10 minutes | **Cook Time:** 0 minutes | **Total Time:** 10 minutes | **Per Serving:** 4 servings

Ingredients:

- 1 apple, sliced
- 1 cup strawberries, halved
- 1 cup blueberries
- 1 cup sliced cucumbers
- 1/2 cup almond butter (unsweetened, low sodium)

Instructions:

1. Arrange the apple slices, strawberries, blueberries, and cucumber slices on a large platter.
2. Serve with a bowl of almond butter for dipping.

Nutritional Value: Calories: 200 | Phosphorus: 80 mg | Sodium: 5 mg | Protein: 5 g | Carbohydrates: 25 g | Fats: 10 g | Potassium: 220 mg | Iron: 1 mg

CKD-Friendly Hummus with Carrot and Celery Sticks

Prep Time: 15 minutes | **Cook Time:** 0 minutes | **Total Time:** 15 minutes | **Per Serving:** 4 servings

Ingredients:

- 1 can (15 ounces) low-sodium chickpeas, drained and rinsed
- 2 tablespoons tahini
- 1 clove garlic, minced
- 2 tablespoons lemon juice
- 2 tablespoons olive oil
- 1/4 cup water
- Salt, to taste
- 2 large carrots, cut into sticks
- 4 celery stalks, cut into sticks

Instructions:

1. In a food processor, combine the chickpeas, tahini, garlic, lemon juice, olive oil, and water. Blend until smooth.
2. Season with salt to taste.
3. Serve the hummus with carrot and celery sticks.

Nutritional Value: Calories: 180 | Phosphorus: 110 mg | Sodium: 80 mg | Protein: 5 g | Carbohydrates: 20 g | Fats: 10 g | Potassium: 250 mg | Iron: 1.5 mg

Roasted Chickpeas Seasoned with Herbs and Spices

Prep Time: 10 minutes | **Cook Time:** 30 minutes | **Total Time:** 40 minutes | **Per Serving:** 4 servings

Ingredients:

- 1 can (15 ounces) low-sodium chickpeas, drained and rinsed
- 1 tablespoon olive oil
- 1 teaspoon paprika
- 1 teaspoon garlic powder
- 1 teaspoon dried oregano
- Salt and pepper, to taste

Instructions:

1. Preheat the oven to 400°F (200°C).
2. Pat the chickpeas dry with a paper towel and place them in a large bowl.
3. Add the olive oil, paprika, garlic powder, oregano, salt, and pepper. Toss until the chickpeas are evenly coated.
4. Spread the chickpeas in a single layer on a baking sheet.
5. Roast for 25-30 minutes, stirring halfway through, until the chickpeas are crispy.
6. Let cool slightly before serving.

Nutritional Value: Calories: 150 | Phosphorus: 110 mg | Sodium: 70 mg | Protein: 5 g | Carbohydrates: 20 g | Fats: 5 g | Potassium: 240 mg | Iron: 2 mg

Low-Sodium Trail Mix with Nuts and Dried Fruit

Prep Time: 5 minutes | **Cook Time:** 0 minutes | **Total Time:** 5 minutes | **Per Serving:** 4 servings

Ingredients:

- 1/2 cup unsalted almonds
- 1/2 cup unsalted cashews
- 1/4 cup dried cranberries (unsweetened)
- 1/4 cup dried blueberries (unsweetened)
- 1/4 cup pumpkin seeds (unsalted)
- 1/4 cup sunflower seeds (unsalted)

Instructions:

1. In a large bowl, combine all the ingredients and mix well.
2. Store in an airtight container.

Nutritional Value: Calories: 200 | Phosphorus: 150 mg | Sodium: 10 mg | Protein: 6 g | Carbohydrates: 20 g | Fats: 12 g | Potassium: 250 mg | Iron: 2 mg

Kidney-friendly guacamole with Whole Wheat Tortilla Chips

Prep Time: 15 minutes | **Cook Time:** 10 minutes | **Total Time:** 25 minutes | **Per Serving:** 4 servings

Ingredients:

- 2 ripe avocados
- 1 small tomato, diced
- 1/4 red onion, finely chopped
- 1 clove garlic, minced
- 1 tablespoon lime juice
- 1 tablespoon fresh cilantro, chopped
- Salt, to taste
- 4 whole wheat tortillas
- 1 tablespoon olive oil

Instructions:

1. Preheat the oven to 350°F (175°C).
2. Cut the tortillas into wedges and place them on a baking sheet. Brush with olive oil.
3. Bake for 10 minutes or until crispy, turning halfway through.
4. Meanwhile, in a bowl, mash the avocados with a fork.
5. Stir in the tomato, onion, garlic, lime juice, cilantro, and salt.
6. Serve the guacamole with the whole wheat tortilla chips.

Nutritional Value: Calories: 250 | Phosphorus: 120 mg | Sodium: 80 mg | Protein: 4 g | Carbohydrates: 30 g | Fats: 15 g | Potassium: 350 mg | Iron: 1.5 mg

Cucumber and Cream Cheese Roll-Ups

Prep Time: 15 minutes | **Cook Time:** 0 minutes | **Total Time:** 15 minutes | **Per Serving:** 4 servings

Ingredients:

- 2 large cucumbers, thinly sliced lengthwise
- 1/2 cup low-fat cream cheese
- 1 tablespoon fresh dill, chopped
- 1 tablespoon fresh chives, chopped
- 1 teaspoon lemon juice
- Salt, to taste

Instructions:

1. In a small bowl, mix the cream cheese, dill, chives, lemon juice, and salt until well combined.
2. Spread a thin layer of the cream cheese mixture onto each cucumber slice.
3. Roll up the cucumber slices and secure with toothpicks if necessary.
4. Serve immediately or refrigerate until ready to serve.

Nutritional Value: Calories: 60 | Phosphorus: 20 mg | Sodium: 45 mg | Protein: 2 g | Carbohydrates: 4 g | Fats: 4 g | Potassium: 100 mg | Iron: 0.2 mg

CKD-Friendly Spinach and Artichoke Dip with Whole Wheat Pita Chips

Prep Time: 15 minutes | **Cook Time:** 20 minutes | **Total Time:** 35 minutes | **Per Serving:** 4 servings

Ingredients:

- 1 cup frozen spinach, thawed and drained
- 1 can (14 ounces) artichoke hearts, drained and chopped
- 1/2 cup low-fat Greek yogurt
- 1/4 cup low-fat cream cheese
- 1/4 cup grated Parmesan cheese
- 1 clove garlic, minced
- 1 teaspoon lemon juice
- Salt and pepper, to taste
- 4 whole wheat pitas, cut into chips
- 1 tablespoon olive oil

Instructions:

1. Preheat the oven to 375°F (190°C).
2. In a bowl, mix the spinach, artichoke hearts, Greek yogurt, cream cheese, Parmesan cheese, garlic, lemon juice, salt, and pepper until well combined.
3. Spread the mixture into a baking dish and bake for 20 minutes, or until bubbly and lightly browned.
4. Meanwhile, brush the pita chips with olive oil and bake for 10-12 minutes, or until crispy.
5. Serve the dip warm with the pita chips.

Nutritional Value: Calories: 220 | Phosphorus: 150 mg | Sodium: 170 mg | Protein: 8 g | Carbohydrates: 30 g | Fats: 8 g | Potassium: 250 mg | Iron: 2 mg

Grilled Vegetable Skewers with Low-Fat Ranch Dip

Prep Time: 20 minutes | **Cook Time:** 15 minutes | **Total Time:** 35 minutes | **Per Serving:** 4 servings

Ingredients:

- 1 red bell pepper, cut into chunks
- 1 yellow bell pepper, cut into chunks
- 1 zucchini, sliced
- 1 red onion, cut into chunks
- 1 tablespoon olive oil
- Salt and pepper, to taste
- 1/2 cup low-fat Greek yogurt
- 2 tablespoons buttermilk
- 1 tablespoon fresh dill, chopped
- 1 tablespoon fresh parsley, chopped
- 1 teaspoon garlic powder
- 1 teaspoon onion powder

Instructions:

1. Preheat the grill to medium heat.
2. Thread the bell peppers, zucchini, and red onion onto skewers.
3. Brush the vegetables with olive oil and season with salt and pepper.
4. Grill the skewers for 10-15 minutes, turning occasionally, until tender and lightly charred.
5. Meanwhile, in a bowl, mix the Greek yogurt, buttermilk, dill, parsley, garlic powder, and onion powder to make the ranch dip.
6. Serve the vegetable skewers with the ranch dip.

Nutritional Value: Calories: 120 | Phosphorus: 90 mg | Sodium: 80 mg | Protein: 4 g | Carbohydrates: 10 g | Fats: 7 g | Potassium: 350 mg | Iron: 0.5 mg

High-Fiber Granola Bars with Dried Fruit and Nuts

Prep Time: 15 minutes | **Cook Time:** 25 minutes | **Total Time:** 40 minutes | **Per Serving:** 8 servings

Ingredients:

- 2 cups rolled oats
- 1/4 cup flaxseeds
- 1/4 cup unsweetened shredded coconut
- 1/4 cup honey or maple syrup
- 1/4 cup almond butter
- 1/4 cup dried cranberries
- 1/4 cup dried blueberries
- 1/4 cup chopped almonds (unsalted)
- 1 teaspoon vanilla extract

Instructions:

1. Preheat the oven to 350°F (175°C).
2. In a large bowl, combine the oats, flaxseeds, and shredded coconut.
3. In a small saucepan, heat the honey (or maple syrup) and almond butter over low heat until melted and smooth.
4. Remove from heat and stir in the vanilla extract.
5. Pour the wet mixture over the dry ingredients and mix until well combined.
6. Stir in the dried cranberries, dried blueberries, and chopped almonds.
7. Press the mixture into a greased 9x9-inch baking pan.
8. Bake for 20-25 minutes, or until golden brown.
9. Let cool completely before cutting into bars.

Nutritional Value: Calories: 210 | Phosphorus: 100 mg | Sodium: 15 mg | Protein: 5 g | Carbohydrates: 30 g | Fats: 9 g | Potassium: 150 mg | Iron: 1 mg

CKD-Friendly Edamame and Cherry Tomato Salad

Prep Time: 10 minutes | **Cook Time:** 5 minutes | **Total Time:** 15 minutes | **Per Serving:** 4 servings

Ingredients:

- 1 cup shelled edamame (fresh or frozen)
- 1 cup cherry tomatoes, halved
- 1/4 cup red onion, finely chopped
- 2 tablespoons olive oil
- 1 tablespoon lemon juice
- 1 teaspoon balsamic vinegar
- Salt and pepper, to taste

Instructions:

1. If using frozen edamame, cook according to package instructions and let cool.
2. In a large bowl, combine the edamame, cherry tomatoes, and red onion.
3. In a small bowl, whisk together the olive oil, lemon juice, balsamic vinegar, salt, and pepper.
4. Pour the dressing over the salad and toss until well combined.
5. Serve immediately.

Nutritional Value: Calories: 150 | Phosphorus: 100 mg | Sodium: 30 mg | Protein: 6 g | Carbohydrates: 12 g | Fats: 10 g | Potassium: 250 mg | Iron: 1 mg

Desserts

Fresh Fruit Salad with a Dollop of Whipped Cream

Prep Time: 10 minutes | **Cook Time:** 0 minutes | **Total Time:** 10 minutes | **Per Serving:** 4 servings

Ingredients:

- 1 cup strawberries, hulled and sliced
- 1 cup blueberries
- 1 cup apple, diced
- 1 cup grapes, halved
- 1 cup pineapple, diced
- 1 cup low-fat whipped cream

Instructions:

1. In a large bowl, combine the strawberries, blueberries, apples, grapes, and pineapple.
2. Gently toss the fruits to mix.
3. Serve the fruit salad in individual bowls, each topped with a dollop of whipped cream.

Nutritional Value: Calories: 90 | Phosphorus: 25 mg | Sodium: 10 mg | Protein: 1 g | Carbohydrates: 20 g | Fats: 2 g | Potassium: 150 mg | Iron: 0.3 mg

CKD-Friendly Chocolate Chip Cookies with Oat Flour

Prep Time: 15 minutes | **Cook Time:** 12 minutes | **Total Time:** 27 minutes | **Per Serving:** 12 servings

Ingredients:

- 1 cup oat flour
- 1/2 teaspoon baking soda
- 1/4 teaspoon salt
- 1/4 cup unsalted butter, softened
- 1/4 cup granulated sugar
- 1/4 cup brown sugar
- 1 large egg
- 1 teaspoon vanilla extract
- 1/2 cup dark chocolate chips (low potassium)

Instructions:

1. Preheat the oven to 350°F (175°C). Line a baking sheet with parchment paper.
2. In a small bowl, combine the oat flour, baking soda, and salt.
3. In a large bowl, beat the butter, granulated sugar, and brown sugar until creamy.
4. Add the egg and vanilla extract, mixing well.
5. Gradually add the dry ingredients to the wet mixture, stirring until combined.
6. Fold in the chocolate chips.
7. Drop spoonfuls of dough onto the prepared baking sheet.
8. Bake for 10-12 minutes or until edges are lightly browned.
9. Allow cookies to cool on the baking sheet for a few minutes before transferring to a wire rack.

Nutritional Value: Calories: 120 | Phosphorus: 35 mg | Sodium: 40 mg | Protein: 2 g | Carbohydrates: 18 g | Fats: 5 g | Potassium: 50 mg | Iron: 0.5 mg

Low-sugar banana Bread with Walnuts and Oat Flour

Prep Time: 15 minutes | **Cook Time:** 50 minutes | **Total Time:** 1 hour 5 minutes | **Per Serving:** 8 servings

Ingredients:

- 1 cup oat flour
- 1/2 cup whole wheat flour
- 1 teaspoon baking soda
- 1/4 teaspoon salt
- 1/4 cup unsalted butter, melted
- 1/4 cup honey
- 2 large eggs
- 1 teaspoon vanilla extract
- 3 ripe bananas, mashed
- 1/4 cup chopped walnuts

Instructions:

1. Preheat the oven to 350°F (175°C). Grease a loaf pan.
2. In a medium bowl, combine the oat flour, whole wheat flour, baking soda, and salt.
3. In a large bowl, mix the melted butter, honey, eggs, and vanilla extract until well combined.
4. Stir in the mashed bananas.
5. Gradually add the dry ingredients to the wet mixture, stirring until just combined.
6. Fold in the chopped walnuts.
7. Pour the batter into the prepared loaf pan.
8. Bake for 50 minutes or until a toothpick inserted into the center comes out clean.
9. Allow the bread to cool in the pan for 10 minutes before transferring to a wire rack.

Nutritional Value: Calories: 180 | Phosphorus: 45 mg | Sodium: 100 mg | Protein: 4 g | Carbohydrates: 28 g | Fats: 7 g | Potassium: 150 mg | Iron: 1 mg

Kidney-Friendly No-Bake Energy Bites with Oats and Peanut Butter

Prep Time: 15 minutes | **Cook Time:** 0 minutes | **Total Time:** 15 minutes | **Per Serving:** 12 servings

Ingredients:

- 1 cup rolled oats
- 1/4 cup peanut butter (unsweetened)
- 1/4 cup honey
- 1/4 cup unsweetened shredded coconut
- 1/4 cup mini dark chocolate chips (low potassium)
- 1 teaspoon vanilla extract

Instructions:

1. In a large bowl, combine the oats, peanut butter, honey, shredded coconut, dark chocolate chips, and vanilla extract.
2. Mix until well combined.
3. Roll the mixture into small balls.
4. Place the energy bites on a baking sheet lined with parchment paper.
5. Refrigerate for at least 30 minutes before serving.

Nutritional Value: Calories: 100 | Phosphorus: 30 mg | Sodium: 20 mg | Protein: 2 g | Carbohydrates: 13 g | Fats: 4 g | Potassium: 60 mg | Iron: 0.5 mg

CKD-Friendly Vanilla Pudding with Fresh Berries and Whipped Cream

Prep Time: 15 minutes | **Cook Time:** 15 minutes | **Total Time:** 30 minutes | **Per Serving:** 4 servings

Ingredients:

- 2 cups low-fat milk
- 1/4 cup granulated sugar
- 3 tablespoons cornstarch
- 1 teaspoon vanilla extract
- 1 cup mixed fresh berries (strawberries, blueberries, raspberries)
- 1/2 cup low-fat whipped cream

Instructions:

1. In a medium saucepan, combine the milk, sugar, and cornstarch.
2. Cook over medium heat, stirring constantly until the mixture thickens and begins to boil.
3. Remove from heat and stir in the vanilla extract.
4. Pour the pudding into individual serving bowls and let cool to room temperature.
5. Refrigerate for at least 2 hours before serving.
6. Serve topped with fresh berries and a dollop of whipped cream.

Nutritional Value: Calories: 160 | Phosphorus: 80 mg | Sodium: 70 mg | Protein: 5 g | Carbohydrates: 29 g | Fats: 2 g | Potassium: 150 mg | Iron: 0.3 mg

Grilled Pineapple with a Dollop of Low-Fat Yogurt

Prep Time: 10 minutes | **Cook Time:** 6 minutes | **Total Time:** 16 minutes | **Per Serving:** 4 servings

Ingredients:

- 1 fresh pineapple, peeled, cored, and cut into rings
- 1 tablespoon honey
- 1/2 teaspoon ground cinnamon
- 1 cup low-fat Greek yogurt

Instructions:

1. Preheat the grill to medium-high heat.
2. In a small bowl, mix the honey and cinnamon.
3. Brush the pineapple rings with the honey mixture.
4. Grill the pineapple rings for 3 minutes on each side, or until grill marks appear.
5. Serve the grilled pineapple with a dollop of low-fat Greek yogurt.

Nutritional Value: Calories: 90 | Phosphorus: 45 mg | Sodium: 20 mg | Protein: 5 g | Carbohydrates: 18 g | Fats: 1 g | Potassium: 180 mg | Iron: 0.4 mg

CKD-Friendly Apple Crisp with Oat Topping and Low-Fat Vanilla Ice Cream

Prep Time: 15 minutes | **Cook Time:** 40 minutes | **Total Time:** 55 minutes | **Per Serving:** 8 servings

Ingredients:

- 4 cups sliced apples (low-potassium variety)
- 1 tablespoon lemon juice
- 1/4 cup granulated sugar
- 1/2 teaspoon ground cinnamon
- 1/2 cup old-fashioned oats
- 1/4 cup oat flour
- 1/4 cup chopped walnuts
- 2 tablespoons unsalted butter, melted
- 2 tablespoons honey
- Low-fat vanilla ice cream, for serving

Instructions:

1. Preheat the oven to 350°F (175°C). Grease an 8-inch square baking dish.
2. In a large bowl, toss the sliced apples with lemon juice, sugar, and cinnamon.
3. Spread the apple mixture evenly in the prepared baking dish.
4. In a separate bowl, combine the oats, oat flour, chopped walnuts, melted butter, and honey. Mix until crumbly.
5. Sprinkle the oat mixture over the apples.
6. Bake for 35-40 minutes, or until the topping is golden brown and the apples are tender.
7. Serve warm with a scoop of low-fat vanilla ice cream.

Nutritional Value: Calories: 180 | Phosphorus: 40 mg | Sodium: 20 mg | Protein: 3 g | Carbohydrates: 30 g | Fats: 6 g | Potassium: 100 mg | Iron: 0.7 mg

Low-sugar carrot Cake with Cream Cheese Frosting

Prep Time: 20 minutes | **Cook Time:** 30 minutes | **Total Time:** 50 minutes | **Per Serving:** 12 servings

Ingredients:

- 2 cups oat flour
- 1 teaspoon baking powder
- 1/2 teaspoon baking soda
- 1/2 teaspoon ground cinnamon
- 1/4 teaspoon ground nutmeg
- 1/4 teaspoon salt
- 2 large eggs
- 1/2 cup unsweetened applesauce
- 1/4 cup honey
- 1/4 cup unsalted butter, melted
- 1 teaspoon vanilla extract
- 1 cup grated carrots
- 1/4 cup chopped walnuts (optional)

Cream Cheese Frosting:

- 4 ounces low-fat cream cheese, softened
- 2 tablespoons unsalted butter, softened
- 1 cup powdered sugar
- 1 teaspoon vanilla extract

Instructions:

1. Preheat the oven to 350°F (175°C). Grease an 8-inch square baking dish.
2. In a large bowl, whisk together the oat flour, baking powder, baking soda, cinnamon, nutmeg, and salt.
3. In another bowl, beat the eggs, applesauce, honey, melted butter, and vanilla extract until well combined.
4. Gradually add the dry ingredients to the wet ingredients, mixing until just combined.
5. Fold in the grated carrots and chopped walnuts.
6. Pour the batter into the prepared baking dish and smooth the top.

7. Bake for 25-30 minutes, or until a toothpick inserted into the center comes out clean.

8. Allow the cake to cool completely before frosting.

Cream Cheese Frosting:

1. In a medium bowl, beat the cream cheese and butter until smooth.

2. Gradually add the powdered sugar and vanilla extract, beating until creamy.

3. Spread the frosting over the cooled cake.

Nutritional Value: Calories: 220 | Phosphorus: 55 mg | Sodium: 90 mg | Protein: 4 g | Carbohydrates: 30 g | Fats: 10 g | Potassium: 100 mg | Iron: 1 mg

CKD-Friendly Chocolate Mousse with Fresh Fruit and Whipped Cream

Prep Time: 15 minutes | **Cook Time:** 10 minutes | **Total Time:** 25 minutes | **Per Serving:** 4 servings

Ingredients:

- 4 ounces low-fat cream cheese, softened
- 1/4 cup unsweetened cocoa powder
- 1/4 cup powdered sugar
- 1 teaspoon vanilla extract
- 1/2 cup low-fat Greek yogurt
- Fresh fruit, for serving
- Low-fat whipped cream, for serving

Instructions:

1. In a mixing bowl, beat the cream cheese until smooth.
2. Add the cocoa powder, powdered sugar, and vanilla extract. Mix until well combined.
3. Gently fold in the Greek yogurt until smooth and creamy.
4. Divide the mousse into serving dishes and refrigerate for at least 1 hour.
5. Serve topped with fresh fruit and a dollop of low-fat whipped cream.

Nutritional Value: Calories: 120 | Phosphorus: 75 mg | Sodium: 80 mg | Protein: 5 g | Carbohydrates: 15 g | Fats: 4 g | Potassium: 150 mg | Iron: 1 mg

Kidney-Friendly Rice Pudding with Cinnamon and Raisins

Prep Time: 5 minutes | **Cook Time:** 25 minutes | **Total Time:** 30 minutes | **Per Serving:** 4 servings

Ingredients:

- 1/2 cup white rice
- 2 cups low-fat milk
- 2 tablespoons granulated sugar
- 1/2 teaspoon ground cinnamon
- 1/4 cup raisins

Instructions:

1. In a saucepan, combine the rice, milk, sugar, and cinnamon.
2. Bring to a boil over medium-high heat.
3. Reduce the heat to low and simmer, uncovered, stirring occasionally, for 20-25 minutes or until the rice is tender and the mixture is creamy.
4. Stir in the raisins and cook for an additional 2-3 minutes.
5. Remove from heat and let cool slightly before serving.

Nutritional Value: Calories: 160 | Phosphorus: 125 mg | Sodium: 70 mg | Protein: 5 g | Carbohydrates: 30 g | Fats: 2 g | Potassium: 180 mg | Iron: 1 mg

CKD-Friendly Rice Pudding with Cinnamon and Raisins

Prep Time: 5 minutes | **Cook Time:** 25 minutes | **Total Time:** 30 minutes | **Per Serving:** 4 servings

Ingredients:

- 1/2 cup white rice
- 2 cups low-fat milk
- 2 tablespoons granulated sugar
- 1/2 teaspoon ground cinnamon
- 1/4 cup raisins

Instructions:

1. In a saucepan, combine the rice, milk, sugar, and cinnamon.
2. Bring to a boil over medium-high heat.
3. Reduce the heat to low and simmer, uncovered, stirring occasionally, for 20-25 minutes or until the rice is tender and the mixture is creamy.
4. Stir in the raisins and cook for an additional 2-3 minutes.
5. Remove from heat and let cool slightly before serving.

Nutritional Value: Calories: 160 | Phosphorus: 125 mg | Sodium: 70 mg | Protein: 5 g | Carbohydrates: 30 g | Fats: 2 g | Potassium: 180 mg | Iron: 1 mg

Beverages

CKD-Friendly Iced Tea with Lemon and Mint

Prep Time: 5 minutes | **Cook Time:** 5 minutes | **Total Time:** 10 minutes | **Per Serving:** 4 servings

Ingredients:

- 4 cups water
- 4 black tea bags
- 1 lemon, thinly sliced
- 1/4 cup fresh mint leaves
- Ice cubes, for serving
- Lemon slices and fresh mint sprigs, for garnish (optional)

Instructions:

1. In a saucepan, bring water to a boil.
2. Remove from heat and add the tea bags, lemon slices, and mint leaves.
3. Let the tea steep for 5 minutes.
4. Remove the tea bags and strain the tea into a pitcher.
5. Refrigerate until chilled.
6. Serve over ice cubes and garnish with lemon slices and fresh mint sprigs if desired.

Nutritional Value: Calories: 0 | Phosphorus: 0 mg | Sodium: 5 mg | Protein: 0 g | Carbohydrates: 0 g | Fats: 0 g | Potassium: 10 mg | Iron: 0 mg

Low-sodium vegetable Juice with a Squeeze of Lemon

Prep Time: 5 minutes | **Cook Time:** 0 minutes | **Total Time:** 5 minutes | **Per Serving:** 1 serving

Ingredients:

- 1 cup low-sodium vegetable juice
- 1/2 lemon, juiced

Instructions:

1. In a glass, pour the low-sodium vegetable juice.
2. Squeeze the lemon juice into the glass and stir to combine.
3. Serve immediately over ice if desired.

Nutritional Value: Calories: 50 | Phosphorus: 20 mg | Sodium: 140 mg | Protein: 2 g | Carbohydrates: 12 g | Fats: 0 g | Potassium: 600 mg | Iron: 2 mg

Kidney-Friendly Infused Water with Cucumber and Mint

Prep Time: 5 minutes | **Cook Time:** 0 minutes | **Total Time:** 5 minutes | **Per Serving:** 1 serving

Ingredients:

- 1 cup water
- 3 cucumber slices
- 2 fresh mint leaves
- Ice cubes, for serving

Instructions:

1. In a glass, add the cucumber slices and mint leaves.
2. Pour water over the cucumber and mint.
3. Let it sit for a few minutes to allow the flavors to infuse.
4. Add ice cubes and serve.

Nutritional Value: Calories: 0 | Phosphorus: 10 mg | Sodium: 0 mg | Protein: 0 g | Carbohydrates: 0 g | Fats: 0 g | Potassium: 50 mg | Iron: 0 mg

CKD-Friendly Herbal Tea with a Splash of Lemon

Prep Time: 5 minutes | **Cook Time:** 5 minutes | **Total Time:** 10 minutes | **Per Serving:** 1 serving

Ingredients:

- 1 herbal tea bag (choose a caffeine-free, herbal tea)
- 1 cup boiling water
- 1/2 lemon, juiced

Instructions:

1. Place the herbal tea bag in a cup and pour boiling water over it.
2. Let it steep for 5 minutes.
3. Remove the tea bag and stir in the lemon juice.
4. Serve hot.

Nutritional Value: Calories: 0 | Phosphorus: 0 mg | Sodium: 5 mg | Protein: 0 g | Carbohydrates: 0 g | Fats: 0 g | Potassium: 10 mg | Iron: 0 mg

Low-calorie hot Chocolate with Almond Milk and Whipped Cream

Prep Time: 5 minutes | **Cook Time:** 5 minutes | **Total Time:** 10 minutes | **Per Serving:** 1 serving

Ingredients:

- 1 cup unsweetened almond milk
- 2 tablespoons unsweetened cocoa powder
- 1 tablespoon granulated sugar (optional)
- 1/4 teaspoon vanilla extract
- Low-fat whipped cream, for serving

Instructions:

1. In a small saucepan, heat the almond milk over medium heat until hot but not boiling.
2. Whisk in the cocoa powder, sugar (if using), and vanilla extract until well combined and smooth.
3. Pour the hot chocolate into a mug.
4. Top with low-fat whipped cream.
5. Serve hot.

Nutritional Value: Calories: 50 | Phosphorus: 60 mg | Sodium: 180 mg | Protein: 1 g | Carbohydrates: 8 g | Fats: 2 g | Potassium: 180 mg | Iron: 0.5 mg

CKD-Friendly Fresh Lemonade with a Twist of Lime

Prep Time: 10 minutes | **Cook Time:** 0 minutes | **Total Time:** 10 minutes | **Per Serving:** 1 serving

Ingredients:

- 1 cup water
- 1 lemon, juiced
- 1/2 lime, juiced
- 1 tablespoon granulated sugar (optional)
- Ice cubes, for serving
- Lemon and lime slices, for garnish (optional)
- Fresh mint leaves, for garnish (optional)

Instructions:

1. In a glass, combine the water, lemon juice, lime juice, and sugar (if using). Stir until the sugar is dissolved.
2. Add ice cubes to the glass.
3. Garnish with lemon and lime slices and fresh mint leaves if desired.
4. Stir well before serving.

Nutritional Value: Calories: 10 | Phosphorus: 10 mg | Sodium: 5 mg | Protein: 0 g | Carbohydrates: 3 g | Fats: 0 g | Potassium: 30 mg | Iron: 0 mg

Kidney-Friendly Sparkling Water with a Squeeze of Lemon

Prep Time: 5 minutes | **Cook Time:** 0 minutes | **Total Time:** 5 minutes | **Per Serving:** 1 serving

Ingredients:

- 1 cup sparkling water
- 1/2 lemon, juiced

Instructions:

1. In a glass, pour the sparkling water.
2. Squeeze the lemon juice into the glass and stir to combine.
3. Serve immediately over ice if desired.

Nutritional Value: Calories: 0 | Phosphorus: 0 mg | Sodium: 0 mg | Protein: 0 g | Carbohydrates: 0 g | Fats: 0 g | Potassium: 0 mg | Iron: 0 mg

CKD-Friendly Cranberry Juice with a Splash of Water

Prep Time: 5 minutes | **Cook Time:** 0 minutes | **Total Time:** 5 minutes | **Per Serving:** 1 serving

Ingredients:

- 3/4 cup unsweetened cranberry juice
- 1/4 cup water
- Ice cubes, for serving

Instructions:

1. In a glass, combine the cranberry juice and water.
2. Add ice cubes to the glass and stir well.
3. Serve immediately.

Nutritional Value: Calories: 20 | Phosphorus: 5 mg | Sodium: 5 mg | Protein: 0 g | Carbohydrates: 5 g | Fats: 0 g | Potassium: 10 mg | Iron: 0 mg

Low-sodium tomato Juice with a Splash of Lemon

Prep Time: 5 minutes | **Cook Time:** 0 minutes | **Total Time:** 5 minutes | **Per Serving:** 1 serving

Ingredients:

- 1 cup low-sodium tomato juice
- 1/2 lemon, juiced

Instructions:

1. In a glass, pour the low-sodium tomato juice.
2. Squeeze the lemon juice into the glass and stir to combine.
3. Serve immediately over ice if desired.

Nutritional Value: Calories: 20 | Phosphorus: 50 mg | Sodium: 60 mg | Protein: 1 g | Carbohydrates: 5 g | Fats: 0 g | Potassium: 220 mg | Iron: 1 mg

CKD-Friendly Ginger Ale with a Squeeze of Lime

Prep Time: 5 minutes | **Cook Time:** 0 minutes | **Total Time:** 5 minutes | **Per Serving:** 1 serving

Ingredients:

- 1 cup ginger ale (low sodium, if available)
- 1/2 lime, juiced

Instructions:

1. In a glass, pour the ginger ale.
2. Squeeze the lime juice into the glass and stir to combine.
3. Serve immediately over ice if desired.

Nutritional Value: Calories: 60 | Phosphorus: 0 mg | Sodium: 15 mg | Protein: 0 g | Carbohydrates: 15 g | Fats: 0 g | Potassium: 10 mg | Iron: 0 mg

Chapter 8: Special Diet Considerations

Diabetic-Friendly Recipes

Low-Sugar Blueberry Oat Muffins

Prep Time: 10 minutes | **Cook Time:** 20 minutes | **Total Time:** 30 minutes | **Per Serving:** 12 servings

Ingredients:

- 1 1/2 cups oat flour
- 1/2 cup rolled oats
- 2 teaspoons baking powder
- 1/2 teaspoon baking soda
- 1/4 teaspoon salt
- 1/2 cup unsweetened applesauce
- 1/4 cup honey or maple syrup
- 1/4 cup unsweetened almond milk
- 2 eggs
- 1 teaspoon vanilla extract
- 1 cup fresh or frozen blueberries

Instructions:

1. Preheat the oven to 350°F (175°C). Line a muffin tin with paper liners or grease with cooking spray.
2. In a large bowl, whisk together the oat flour, rolled oats, baking powder, baking soda, and salt.
3. In another bowl, mix the applesauce, honey or maple syrup, almond milk, eggs, and vanilla extract until well combined.
4. Pour the wet ingredients into the dry ingredients and stir until just combined.
5. Gently fold in the blueberries.
6. Divide the batter evenly among the muffin cups, filling each about 3/4 full.
7. Bake for 18-20 minutes, or until a toothpick inserted into the center comes out clean.
8. Allow the muffins to cool in the tin for 5 minutes before transferring to a wire rack to cool completely.

Nutritional Value (per serving): Calories: 120 | Phosphorus: 50 mg | Sodium: 100 mg | Protein: 3 g | Carbohydrates: 20 g | Fats: 3 g | Potassium: 70 mg | Iron: 1 mg

Quinoa and Black Bean Stuffed Peppers

Prep Time: 15 minutes | **Cook Time:** 30 minutes | **Total Time:** 45 minutes | **Per Serving:** 4 servings

Ingredients:

- 4 large bell peppers, any color
- 1 cup cooked quinoa
- 1 cup black beans, drained and rinsed
- 1 cup diced tomatoes
- 1/2 cup corn kernels (fresh, canned, or frozen)
- 1/2 cup diced onion
- 1 clove garlic, minced
- 1 teaspoon ground cumin
- 1/2 teaspoon chili powder
- Salt and pepper, to taste
- 1/2 cup shredded low-fat cheese (optional)
- Fresh cilantro, for garnish

Instructions:

1. Preheat the oven to 375°F (190°C).
2. Cut the tops off the bell peppers and remove the seeds and membranes.
3. In a large bowl, mix the quinoa, black beans, diced tomatoes, corn, onion, garlic, cumin, chili powder, salt, and pepper.
4. Stuff the mixture into the hollowed-out bell peppers.

5. Place the stuffed peppers in a baking dish.

6. If using cheese, sprinkle it over the top of each stuffed pepper.

7. Cover the baking dish with foil and bake for 25 minutes.

8. Remove the foil and bake for an additional 5-10 minutes, or until the peppers are tender and the cheese is melted and bubbly.

9. Garnish with fresh cilantro before serving.

Nutritional Value (per serving without cheese): Calories: 250 | Phosphorus: 100 mg | Sodium: 150 mg | Protein: 10 g | Carbohydrates: 45 g | Fats: 2 g | Potassium: 500 mg | Iron: 3 mg

Grilled Lemon Herb Chicken with Asparagus

Prep Time: 10 minutes | **Cook Time:** 15 minutes | **Total Time:** 25 minutes | **Per Serving:** 4 servings

Ingredients:

- 4 boneless, skinless chicken breasts
- 1 bunch asparagus, woody ends trimmed
- 2 tablespoons olive oil
- 2 cloves garlic, minced
- 2 tablespoons fresh lemon juice
- 1 teaspoon lemon zest
- 1 teaspoon dried oregano
- 1 teaspoon dried thyme
- Salt and pepper, to taste
- Lemon slices, for garnish

Instructions:

1. Preheat the grill to medium-high heat.
2. In a small bowl, whisk together the olive oil, garlic, lemon juice, lemon zest, oregano, thyme, salt, and pepper.
3. Place the chicken breasts and asparagus in a shallow dish and pour the marinade over them.
4. Toss to coat evenly and let marinate for 10 minutes.
5. Remove the chicken and asparagus from the marinade and shake off any excess.
6. Grill the chicken for 6-7 minutes per side, or until cooked through and no longer pink in the center.
7. Grill the asparagus for 3-4 minutes, turning occasionally, until tender and lightly charred.
8. Serve the grilled chicken and asparagus with lemon slices.

Nutritional Value (per serving): Calories: 250 | Phosphorus: 150 mg | Sodium: 100 mg | Protein: 30 g | Carbohydrates: 5 g | Fats: 10 g | Potassium: 400 mg | Iron: 2 mg

Zucchini Noodles with Pesto and Cherry Tomatoes

Prep Time: 15 minutes | **Cook Time:** 5 minutes | **Total Time:** 20 minutes | **Per Serving:** 4 servings

Ingredients:

- 4 medium zucchinis, spiralized into noodles
- 1 cup cherry tomatoes, halved
- 1/4 cup homemade or store-bought pesto
- 2 tablespoons grated Parmesan cheese (optional)
- Salt and pepper, to taste
- Fresh basil leaves, for garnish

Instructions:

1. Heat a large skillet over medium heat.
2. Add the zucchini noodles and cherry tomatoes to the skillet.
3. Cook for 3-5 minutes, or until the zucchini noodles are just tender.
4. Remove from heat and stir in the pesto until well combined.
5. Season with salt and pepper to taste.
6. Divide the zucchini noodles among serving plates.
7. Garnish with grated Parmesan cheese (if using) and fresh basil leaves.

Nutritional Value (per serving without Parmesan cheese): Calories: 100 | Phosphorus: 80 mg | Sodium: 150 mg | Protein: 5 g | Carbohydrates: 10 g | Fats: 5 g | Potassium: 600 mg | Iron: 2 mg

Salmon and Avocado Salad with Citrus Dressing

Prep Time: 10 minutes | **Cook Time:** 10 minutes | **Total Time:** 20 minutes | **Per Serving:** 2 servings

Ingredients:

- 2 salmon fillets
- Salt and pepper, to taste
- 4 cups mixed salad greens
- 1 avocado, sliced
- 1/2 cup cherry tomatoes, halved
- 1/4 cup red onion, thinly sliced
- 1/4 cup sliced almonds
- 2 tablespoons chopped fresh parsley

Citrus Dressing:

- 2 tablespoons fresh lemon juice
- 1 tablespoon fresh orange juice
- 1 tablespoon olive oil
- 1 teaspoon honey or maple syrup
- Salt and pepper, to taste

Instructions:

1. Season the salmon fillets with salt and pepper.
2. Heat a non-stick skillet over medium-high heat. Add the salmon fillets, skin side down, and cook for 4-5 minutes. Flip the fillets and cook for an additional 3-4 minutes, or until cooked through.
3. In a large bowl, combine the mixed salad greens, avocado slices, cherry tomatoes, red onion, sliced almonds, and chopped parsley.

4. In a small bowl, whisk together the lemon juice, orange juice, olive oil, honey or maple syrup, salt, and pepper to make the citrus dressing.

5. Pour the dressing over the salad and toss to coat evenly.

6. Divide the salad between two plates and top each with a salmon fillet.

7. Serve immediately.

Nutritional Value (per serving): Calories: 350 | Phosphorus: 200 mg | Sodium: 150 mg | Protein: 20 g | Carbohydrates: 15 g | Fats: 25 g | Potassium: 600 mg | Iron: 2 mg

Turkey and Vegetable Stir-Fry with Brown Rice

Prep Time: 15 minutes | **Cook Time:** 15 minutes | **Total Time:** 30 minutes | **Per Serving:** 4 servings

Ingredients:

- 1 tablespoon olive oil
- 1-pound lean ground turkey
- 2 cups mixed vegetables (bell peppers, broccoli, snap peas, carrots), sliced
- 2 cloves garlic, minced
- 2 tablespoons low-sodium soy sauce
- 1 tablespoon hoisin sauce
- 1 teaspoon sesame oil
- 2 cups cooked brown rice
- Green onions, sliced, for garnish (optional)
- Sesame seeds, for garnish (optional)

Instructions:

1. Heat olive oil in a large skillet or wok over medium-high heat.
2. Add the ground turkey and cook until browned, breaking it apart with a spoon, about 5-7 minutes.
3. Add the mixed vegetables and minced garlic to the skillet. Cook, stirring frequently, for 3-5 minutes, or until the vegetables are tender-crisp.
4. In a small bowl, whisk together the soy sauce, hoisin sauce, and sesame oil.
5. Pour the sauce over the turkey and vegetable mixture into the skillet. Stir to combine and cook for another 2-3 minutes.
6. Serve the turkey and vegetable stir-fry over cooked brown rice.
7. Garnish with sliced green onions and sesame seeds if desired.

Nutritional Value (per serving): Calories: 350 | Phosphorus: 200 mg | Sodium: 250 mg | Protein: 25 g | Carbohydrates: 35 g | Fats: 12 g | Potassium: 350 mg | Iron: 3 mg

Cauliflower Crust Pizza with Fresh Vegetables

Prep Time: 20 minutes | **Cook Time:** 25 minutes | **Total Time:** 45 minutes | **Per Serving:** 4 servings

Ingredients:

- 1 medium head cauliflower, riced (about 4 cups)
- 1/2 cup grated low-fat mozzarella cheese
- 1/4 cup grated Parmesan cheese
- 1 teaspoon dried oregano
- 1 teaspoon dried basil
- 1/2 teaspoon garlic powder
- 1/4 teaspoon salt
- 1/4 teaspoon black pepper
- 1 egg, beaten
- 1/2 cup tomato sauce (low sodium)
- 1 cup assorted fresh vegetables (bell peppers, cherry tomatoes, mushrooms, red onion), sliced
- 1/4 cup shredded low-fat mozzarella cheese
- Fresh basil leaves, for garnish

Instructions:

1. Preheat the oven to 425°F (220°C). Line a baking sheet with parchment paper.
2. Place the riced cauliflower in a microwave-safe bowl and microwave on high for 4-5 minutes, or until softened.
3. Allow the cauliflower to cool slightly, then transfer it to a clean kitchen towel. Squeeze out as much liquid as possible.
4. In a large bowl, combine the cauliflower, grated mozzarella cheese, Parmesan cheese, dried oregano, dried basil, garlic powder, salt, pepper, and beaten egg. Mix until well combined.
5. Transfer the cauliflower mixture to the prepared baking sheet and shape it into a circle, about 1/4 inch thick.
6. Bake in the preheated oven for 20-25 minutes, or until the crust is golden brown and set.
7. Remove the crust from the oven and spread the tomato sauce evenly over the surface.

8. Arrange the sliced vegetables on top of the sauce and sprinkle with shredded mozzarella cheese.
9. Return the pizza to the oven and bake for an additional 5-7 minutes, or until the cheese is melted and bubbly.
10. Garnish with fresh basil leaves before serving.

Nutritional Value (per serving): Calories: 180 | Phosphorus: 150 mg | Sodium: 200 mg | Protein: 12 g | Carbohydrates: 15 g | Fats: 8 g | Potassium: 300 mg | Iron: 2 mg

Chia Seed Pudding with Mixed Berries

Prep Time: 5 minutes | **Cook Time:** 0 minutes | **Total Time:** 4 hours 5 minutes | **Per Serving:** 2 servings

Ingredients:

- 1/4 cup chia seeds
- 1 cup unsweetened almond milk
- 1 tablespoon honey or maple syrup (optional)
- 1/2 teaspoon vanilla extract
- 1 cup mixed berries (strawberries, blueberries, raspberries)

Instructions:

1. In a mixing bowl, whisk together the chia seeds, almond milk, honey, or maple syrup (if using), and vanilla extract.
2. Let the mixture sit for 5 minutes, then whisk again to prevent clumps from forming.
3. Cover the bowl and refrigerate for at least 4 hours or overnight, until the pudding has thickened.
4. Stir the pudding well before serving.
5. Divide the chia seed pudding between two serving bowls and top with mixed berries.
6. Serve chilled.

Nutritional Value (per serving): Calories: 150 | Phosphorus: 100 mg | Sodium: 50 mg | Protein: 5 g | Carbohydrates: 20 g | Fats: 6 g | Potassium: 200 mg | Iron: 2 mg

Eggplant Parmesan with Whole Wheat Pasta

Prep Time: 20 minutes | **Cook Time:** 40 minutes | **Total Time:** 1 hour | **Per Serving:** 4 servings

Ingredients:

- 1 large eggplant, thinly sliced
- 1 cup whole wheat bread crumbs
- 1/4 cup grated Parmesan cheese
- 1 teaspoon dried oregano
- 1 teaspoon dried basil
- 1/2 teaspoon garlic powder
- 1/4 teaspoon salt
- 1/4 teaspoon black pepper
- 2 eggs, beaten
- 2 cups low-sodium marinara sauce
- 1 cup shredded low-fat mozzarella cheese
- 8 ounces whole wheat spaghetti, cooked according to package instructions
- Fresh basil leaves, for garnish

Instructions:

1. Preheat the oven to 375°F (190°C).
2. In a shallow dish, combine the whole wheat bread crumbs, grated Parmesan cheese, dried oregano, dried basil, garlic powder, salt, and black pepper.
3. Dip each eggplant slice into the beaten eggs, then dredge in the breadcrumb mixture, pressing gently to adhere.

4. Place the coated eggplant slices in a single layer on a baking sheet lined with parchment paper.

5. Bake in the preheated oven for 20-25 minutes, or until golden brown and crispy.

6. Spread a thin layer of marinara sauce on the bottom of a baking dish.

7. Arrange half of the baked eggplant slices in the baking dish.

8. Top with half of the remaining marinara sauce and half of the shredded mozzarella cheese.

9. Repeat the layers with the remaining eggplant slices, marinara sauce, and mozzarella cheese.

10. Bake for an additional 20 minutes, or until the cheese is melted and bubbly. 11. While the eggplant parmesan is baking, cook the whole wheat spaghetti according to the package instructions.

12. Serve the eggplant parmesan with whole wheat spaghetti and garnish with fresh basil leaves.

Nutritional Value (per serving): Calories: 350 | Phosphorus: 250 mg | Sodium: 300 mg | Protein: 15 g | Carbohydrates: 45 g | Fats: 10 g | Potassium: 350 mg | Iron: 3 mg

Greek Yogurt Parfait with Almonds and Berries

Prep Time: 10 minutes | **Cook Time:** 0 minutes | **Total Time:** 10 minutes | **Per Serving:** 1 serving

Ingredients:

- 1/2 cup low-fat Greek yogurt
- 1/4 cup mixed berries (strawberries, blueberries, raspberries)
- 1 tablespoon sliced almonds
- 1 teaspoon honey or maple syrup (optional)

Instructions:

1. In a serving glass or bowl, layer the Greek yogurt, mixed berries, and sliced almonds.
2. Drizzle with honey or maple syrup if desired.
3. Serve immediately.

Nutritional Value (per serving): Calories: 150 | Phosphorus: 150 mg | Sodium: 50 mg | Protein: 15 g | Carbohydrates: 15 g | Fats: 5 g | Potassium: 200 mg | Iron: 1 mg

Low-Sodium Recipes for Hypertension

Lemon Herb Baked Cod with Steamed Green Beans

Prep Time: 10 minutes | **Cook Time:** 15 minutes | **Total Time:** 25 minutes | **Per Serving:** 2 servings

Ingredients:

- 2 cod fillets (4-6 ounces each)
- 1 tablespoon olive oil
- 1 lemon, thinly sliced
- 2 cloves garlic, minced
- 1 teaspoon dried thyme
- 1 teaspoon dried rosemary
- Salt and pepper, to taste
- 1 cup green beans, trimmed
- Lemon wedges, for serving

Instructions:

1. Preheat the oven to 400°F (200°C).
2. Place the cod fillets on a baking sheet lined with parchment paper.
3. Drizzle the cod fillets with olive oil and sprinkle with minced garlic, dried thyme, dried rosemary, salt, and pepper.
4. Arrange lemon slices on top of the cod fillets.
5. Bake in the preheated oven for 12-15 minutes, or until the fish flakes easily with a fork.
6. While the cod is baking, steam the green beans until tender-crisp, about 5-7 minutes.
7. Serve the baked cod with steamed green beans and lemon wedges.

Nutritional Value (per serving): Calories: 200 | Phosphorus: 150 mg | Sodium: 100 mg | Protein: 25 g | Carbohydrates: 5 g | Fats: 8 g | Potassium: 300 mg | Iron: 2 mg

Vegetarian Chili with Kidney Beans and Corn

Prep Time: 10 minutes | **Cook Time:** 30 minutes | **Total Time:** 40 minutes | **Per Serving:** 4 servings

Ingredients:

- 1 tablespoon olive oil
- 1 onion, diced
- 2 cloves garlic, minced
- 1 bell pepper, diced
- 1 zucchini, diced
- 1 can (15 ounces) low-sodium kidney beans, drained and rinsed
- 1 can (15 ounces) low-sodium corn, drained
- 1 can (15 ounces) low sodium diced tomatoes
- 2 cups low-sodium vegetable broth
- 2 teaspoons chili powder
- 1 teaspoon ground cumin
- 1/2 teaspoon paprika
- Salt and pepper, to taste
- Fresh cilantro, chopped, for garnish (optional)

Instructions:

1. Heat olive oil in a large pot over medium heat.
2. Add the diced onion and minced garlic to the pot. Cook, stirring frequently, until the onion is translucent, about 3-4 minutes.
3. Add the diced bell pepper and zucchini to the pot. Cook for another 3-4 minutes, or until the vegetables are slightly softened.
4. Stir in the kidney beans, corn, diced tomatoes, vegetable broth, chili powder, cumin, paprika, salt, and pepper.
5. Bring the chili to a simmer, then reduce the heat to low. Cover and let it simmer for 20-25 minutes, stirring occasionally.
6. Taste and adjust seasoning if necessary.
7. Serve the vegetarian chili hot, garnished with chopped fresh cilantro if desired.

Nutritional Value (per serving): Calories: 250 | Phosphorus: 200 mg | Sodium: 150 mg | Protein: 10 g | Carbohydrates: 40 g | Fats: 5 g | Potassium: 400 mg | Iron: 2 mg

Roasted Garlic and Rosemary Chicken with Mashed Cauliflower

Prep Time: 10 minutes | **Cook Time:** 40 minutes | **Total Time:** 50 minutes | **Per Serving:** 2 servings

Ingredients:

- 2 boneless, skinless chicken breasts
- 2 cloves garlic, minced
- 1 tablespoon fresh rosemary, chopped
- 1 tablespoon olive oil
- Salt and pepper, to taste
- 1 medium head cauliflower, cut into florets
- 2 tablespoons low-fat milk
- 1 tablespoon unsalted butter (optional)

Instructions:

1. Preheat the oven to 400°F (200°C).
2. Place the chicken breasts in a baking dish.
3. In a small bowl, mix the minced garlic, chopped rosemary, olive oil, salt, and pepper.
4. Rub the garlic-rosemary mixture evenly over the chicken breasts.
5. Roast in the preheated oven for 25-30 minutes, or until the chicken is cooked through and no longer pink in the center.
6. While the chicken is roasting, steam the cauliflower florets until tender, about 10-12 minutes.
7. Transfer the steamed cauliflower to a food processor. Add the low-fat milk and unsalted butter (if using).
8. Pulse until smooth and creamy. Season with salt and pepper to taste.
9. Serve the roasted garlic and rosemary chicken with mashed cauliflower.

Nutritional Value (per serving): Calories: 250 | Phosphorus: 200 mg | Sodium: 100 mg | Protein: 30 g | Carbohydrates: 10 g | Fats: 10 g | Potassium: 400 mg | Iron: 2 mg

Spinach and Feta Stuffed Turkey Meatballs

Prep Time: 15 minutes | **Cook Time:** 20 minutes | **Total Time:** 35 minutes | **Per Serving:** 4 servings

Ingredients:

- 1-pound lean ground turkey
- 1/4 cup breadcrumbs (low sodium)
- 1 egg
- 1/4 cup crumbled feta cheese
- 1 cup fresh spinach, chopped
- 2 cloves garlic, minced
- 1 teaspoon dried oregano
- 1/2 teaspoon dried thyme
- Salt and pepper, to taste
- Olive oil cooking spray

Instructions:

1. Preheat the oven to 400°F (200°C).
2. In a large mixing bowl, combine the ground turkey, breadcrumbs, egg, crumbled feta cheese, chopped spinach, minced garlic, dried oregano, dried thyme, salt, and pepper. Mix until well combined.
3. Shape the turkey mixture into meatballs, about 1 inch in diameter.
4. Place the meatballs on a baking sheet lined with parchment paper.
5. Spray the meatballs lightly with olive oil cooking spray.
6. Bake in the preheated oven for 18-20 minutes, or until cooked through and golden brown.
7. Serve the spinach and feta stuffed turkey meatballs with your favorite low-sodium marinara sauce or tzatziki sauce.

Nutritional Value (per serving): Calories: 200 | Phosphorus: 150 mg | Sodium: 100 mg | Protein: 25 g | Carbohydrates: 5 g | Fats: 8 g | Potassium: 300 mg | Iron: 2 mg

Sesame Ginger Tofu Stir-Fry with Bok Choy

Prep Time: 15 minutes | **Cook Time:** 15 minutes | **Total Time:** 30 minutes | **Per Serving:** 2 servings

Ingredients:

- 1 block (14 ounces) extra-firm tofu, drained and cubed
- 2 tablespoons low-sodium soy sauce
- 1 tablespoon rice vinegar
- 1 tablespoon sesame oil
- 1 tablespoon honey
- 1 tablespoon grated ginger
- 2 cloves garlic, minced
- 1 tablespoon cornstarch
- 2 tablespoons water
- 1 tablespoon olive oil
- 2 cups Bok choy, chopped
- 1 bell pepper, sliced
- 1 cup snow peas
- Cooked brown rice, for serving

Instructions:

1. In a small bowl, whisk together the low-sodium soy sauce, rice vinegar, sesame oil, honey, grated ginger, and minced garlic.
2. In another small bowl, mix the cornstarch and water to make a slurry.
3. Heat olive oil in a large skillet or wok over medium-high heat.
4. Add the cubed tofu to the skillet and cook until golden brown on all sides, about 5-7 minutes.
5. Add the Bok choy, sliced bell pepper, and snow peas to the skillet. Cook for another 3-4 minutes, or until the vegetables are tender-crisp.
6. Pour the sauce over the tofu and vegetables in the skillet.
7. Stir in the cornstarch slurry and cook for 1-2 minutes, or until the sauce has thickened.
8. Serve the sesame ginger tofu stir-fry over cooked brown rice.

Nutritional Value (per serving): Calories: 300 | Phosphorus: 200 mg | Sodium: 150 mg | Protein: 15 g | Carbohydrates: 25 g | Fats: 15 g | Potassium: 400 mg | Iron: 3 mg

Quinoa Salad with Cucumber, Tomato, and Feta

Prep Time: 15 minutes | **Cook Time:** 15 minutes | **Total Time:** 30 minutes | **Per Serving:** 4 servings

Ingredients:

- 1 cup quinoa, rinsed
- 2 cups water
- 1 cucumber, diced
- 1 cup cherry tomatoes, halved
- 1/4 cup crumbled feta cheese
- 2 tablespoons fresh parsley, chopped
- 2 tablespoons fresh mint, chopped
- 2 tablespoons extra virgin olive oil
- 1 tablespoon lemon juice
- Salt and pepper, to taste

Instructions:

1. In a medium saucepan, bring the water to a boil.
2. Add the quinoa to the boiling water. Reduce the heat to low, cover, and simmer for 15 minutes, or until the quinoa is tender and the water is absorbed.
3. Remove the quinoa from the heat and let it cool to room temperature.
4. In a large bowl, combine the cooked quinoa, diced cucumber, cherry tomatoes, crumbled feta cheese, chopped parsley, and chopped mint.
5. In a small bowl, whisk together the extra virgin olive oil, lemon juice, salt, and pepper.
6. Pour the dressing over the quinoa salad and toss to combine.
7. Serve the quinoa salad immediately or refrigerate until ready to serve.

Nutritional Value (per serving): Calories: 200 | Phosphorus: 150 mg | Sodium: 100 mg | Protein: 5 g | Carbohydrates: 30 g | Fats: 8 g | Potassium: 200 mg | Iron: 2 mg

Grilled Lemon Dill Shrimp Skewers with Quinoa

Prep Time: 20 minutes | **Cook Time:** 10 minutes | **Total Time:** 30 minutes | **Per Serving:** 2 servings

Ingredients:

- 12 large shrimp, peeled and deveined
- 1 tablespoon olive oil
- 1 tablespoon lemon juice
- 1 teaspoon dried dill
- Salt and pepper, to taste
- 1/2 cup quinoa, rinsed
- 1 cup water
- Lemon wedges, for serving

Instructions:

1. In a bowl, toss the shrimp with olive oil, lemon juice, dried dill, salt, and pepper until evenly coated. Let marinate for 10-15 minutes.
2. Meanwhile, in a medium saucepan, bring the water to a boil. Add the quinoa, reduce the heat to low, cover, and simmer for 15 minutes, or until the quinoa is tender and the water is absorbed. Remove from heat and let it sit for 5 minutes.
3. Preheat the grill to medium-high heat.
4. Thread the marinated shrimp onto skewers.
5. Grill the shrimp skewers for 2-3 minutes per side, or until cooked through and slightly charred.
6. Fluff the cooked quinoa with a fork and divide it between plates.
7. Serve the grilled lemon dill shrimp skewers over quinoa with lemon wedges on the side.

Nutritional Value (per serving): Calories: 250 | Phosphorus: 150 mg | Sodium: 100 mg | Protein: 20 g | Carbohydrates: 20 g | Fats: 10 g | Potassium: 200 mg | Iron: 2 mg

Mushroom and Spinach Risotto with Arborio Rice

Prep Time: 10 minutes | **Cook Time:** 30 minutes | **Total Time:** 40 minutes | **Per Serving:** 2 servings

Ingredients:

- 1 tablespoon olive oil
- 1/2 onion, finely chopped
- 2 cloves garlic, minced
- 1 cup Arborio rice
- 1/4 cup dry white wine (optional)
- 3 cups low-sodium vegetable broth
- 1 cup mushrooms, sliced
- 2 cups baby spinach
- 1/4 cup grated Parmesan cheese
- Salt and pepper, to taste

Instructions:

1. In a medium saucepan, heat the olive oil over medium heat.
2. Add the chopped onion and minced garlic to the saucepan. Cook, stirring occasionally, until the onion is soft and translucent, about 3-4 minutes.
3. Add the Arborio rice to the saucepan. Cook, stirring constantly, for 1-2 minutes, or until the rice is lightly toasted.
4. If using, pour in the dry white wine. Cook, stirring constantly, until the wine is absorbed.
5. Begin adding the vegetable broth to the rice, 1/2 cup at a time, stirring constantly and allowing each addition to be absorbed before adding more. Continue this process until the rice is creamy and tender, about 20-25 minutes.
6. In the last 5 minutes of cooking, stir in the sliced mushrooms and baby spinach.
7. Once the risotto is creamy and the vegetables are tender, remove the saucepan from the heat.
8. Stir in the grated Parmesan cheese and season with salt and pepper to taste.
9. Serve the mushroom and spinach risotto immediately.

Nutritional Value (per serving): Calories: 300 | Phosphorus: 200 mg | Sodium: 100 mg | Protein: 8 g | Carbohydrates: 50 g | Fats: 8 g | Potassium: 250 mg | Iron: 2 mg

Cabbage and Carrot Slaw with Apple Cider Vinaigrette

Prep Time: 10 minutes | **Cook Time:** 0 minutes | **Total Time:** 10 minutes | **Per Serving:** 4 servings

Ingredients:

- 2 cups green cabbage, shredded
- 1 cup carrots, grated
- 2 tablespoons apple cider vinegar
- 1 tablespoon olive oil
- 1 teaspoon honey
- 1 teaspoon Dijon mustard
- Salt and pepper, to taste
- Fresh parsley, chopped, for garnish (optional)

Instructions:

1. In a large bowl, combine the shredded green cabbage and grated carrots.
2. In a small bowl, whisk together the apple cider vinegar, olive oil, honey, Dijon mustard, salt, and pepper to make the vinaigrette.
3. Pour the vinaigrette over the cabbage and carrot mixture. Toss until well coated.
4. Garnish with chopped fresh parsley, if desired.
5. Serve the cabbage and carrot slaw immediately or refrigerate until ready to serve.

Nutritional Value (per serving): Calories: 50 | Phosphorus: 50 mg | Sodium: 50 mg | Protein: 1 g | Carbohydrates: 7 g | Fats: 3 g | Potassium: 150 mg | Iron: 1 mg

Lentil and Vegetable Soup with Herbs

Prep Time: 10 minutes | **Cook Time:** 40 minutes | **Total Time:** 50 minutes | **Per Serving:** 4 servings

Ingredients:

- 1 tablespoon olive oil
- 1 onion, diced
- 2 carrots, diced
- 2 celery stalks, diced
- 2 cloves garlic, minced
- 1 cup dry green lentils, rinsed
- 4 cups low-sodium vegetable broth
- 1 can (14 ounces) diced tomatoes, with juices
- 1 teaspoon dried thyme
- 1 teaspoon dried oregano
- 1 bay leaf
- Salt and pepper, to taste
- 2 cups fresh spinach leaves
- Fresh parsley, chopped, for garnish (optional)

Instructions:

1. In a large pot, heat the olive oil over medium heat.
2. Add the diced onion, carrots, and celery to the pot. Cook, stirring occasionally, until the vegetables are softened, about 5 minutes.
3. Add the minced garlic to the pot and cook for an additional 1-2 minutes, or until fragrant.
4. Stir in the dry green lentils, vegetable broth, diced tomatoes (with juices), dried thyme, dried oregano, bay leaf, salt, and pepper.

5. Bring the soup to a boil, then reduce the heat to low. Cover and simmer for 30 minutes, or until the lentils are tender.

6. Stir in the fresh spinach leaves and cook for an additional 5 minutes, or until the spinach is wilted.

7. Remove the bay leaf from the soup.

8. Taste and adjust the seasoning if necessary.

9. Serve the lentil and vegetable soup hot, garnished with chopped fresh parsley, if desired.

Nutritional Value (per serving): Calories: 200 | Phosphorus: 100 mg | Sodium: 150 mg | Protein: 10 g | Carbohydrates: 30 g | Fats: 3 g | Potassium: 300 mg | Iron: 3 mg

Vegetarian CKD Recipes

Black Bean and Sweet Potato Tacos with Avocado

Prep Time: 15 minutes | **Cook Time:** 25 minutes | **Total Time:** 40 minutes | **Per Serving:** 4 servings

Ingredients:

- 1 tablespoon olive oil
- 1 onion, diced
- 2 cloves garlic, minced
- 1 sweet potato, peeled and diced
- 1 can (15 ounces) black beans, drained and rinsed
- 1 teaspoon ground cumin
- 1 teaspoon chili powder
- 1/2 teaspoon paprika
- Salt and pepper, to taste
- 8 small corn tortillas
- 1 avocado, sliced
- Fresh cilantro, chopped, for garnish
- Lime wedges, for serving

Instructions:

1. Heat olive oil in a large skillet over medium heat.
2. Add the diced onion and minced garlic to the skillet. Cook, stirring occasionally, until the onion is soft and translucent, about 3-4 minutes.
3. Add the diced sweet potato to the skillet. Cook, stirring occasionally, until the sweet potato is tender, about 10-12 minutes.
4. Stir in the black beans, ground cumin, chili powder, paprika, salt, and pepper. Cook for an additional 2-3 minutes, or until heated through.
5. Warm the corn tortillas in a dry skillet or the microwave.
6. Spoon the black bean and sweet potato mixture onto the warm tortillas.
7. Top each taco with sliced avocado and chopped fresh cilantro.
8. Serve the black bean and sweet potato tacos with lime wedges on the side.

Nutritional Value (per serving): Calories: 250 | Phosphorus: 150 mg | Sodium: 100 mg | Protein: 8 g | Carbohydrates: 35 g | Fats: 10 g | Potassium: 300 mg | Iron: 2 mg

Chickpea and Spinach Curry with Basmati Rice

Prep Time: 10 minutes | **Cook Time:** 25 minutes | **Total Time:** 35 minutes | **Per Serving:** 4 servings

Ingredients:

- 1 tablespoon olive oil
- 1 onion, diced
- 2 cloves garlic, minced
- 1 tablespoon grated ginger
- 1 tablespoon curry powder
- 1 teaspoon ground cumin
- 1 teaspoon ground coriander
- 1/2 teaspoon turmeric
- 1 can (15 ounces) chickpeas, drained and rinsed
- 1 can (14 ounces) diced tomatoes
- 1 cup low-sodium vegetable broth
- 4 cups fresh spinach leaves
- Cooked basmati rice, for serving

Instructions:

1. Heat olive oil in a large skillet over medium heat.
2. Add the diced onion to the skillet. Cook, stirring occasionally, until the onion is soft and translucent, about 3-4 minutes.
3. Add the minced garlic and grated ginger to the skillet. Cook for an additional 1-2 minutes, or until fragrant.
4. Stir in the curry powder, ground cumin, ground coriander, and turmeric. Cook for 1 minute, stirring constantly.
5. Add the chickpeas, diced tomatoes (with juices), and low-sodium vegetable broth to the skillet. Bring to a simmer and cook for 10-15 minutes, or until the sauce has thickened slightly.
6. Stir in the fresh spinach leaves and cook for an additional 2-3 minutes, or until the spinach is wilted.
7. Taste and adjust the seasoning if necessary.
8. Serve the chickpea and spinach curry over cooked basmati rice.

Nutritional Value (per serving): Calories: 300 | Phosphorus: 200 mg | Sodium: 100 mg | Protein: 10 g | Carbohydrates: 45 g | Fats: 8 g | Potassium: 400 mg | Iron: 3 mg

Lentil and Vegetable Shepherd's Pie

Prep Time: 20 minutes | **Cook Time:** 40 minutes | **Total Time:** 60 minutes | **Per Serving:** 4 servings

Ingredients:

- 1 tablespoon olive oil
- 1 onion, diced
- 2 carrots, diced
- 2 celery stalks, diced
- 2 cloves garlic, minced
- 1 cup dry green lentils, rinsed
- 2 cups low-sodium vegetable broth
- 1 can (14 ounces) diced tomatoes
- 1 teaspoon dried thyme
- 1 teaspoon dried rosemary
- 1/2 teaspoon paprika
- Salt and pepper, to taste
- 2 cups mashed potatoes (prepared without added salt)
- Fresh parsley, chopped, for garnish (optional)

Instructions:

1. Preheat the oven to 375°F (190°C).
2. Heat olive oil in a large skillet over medium heat.

3. Add the diced onion, carrots, and celery to the skillet. Cook, stirring occasionally, until the vegetables are softened, about 5 minutes.

4. Add the minced garlic to the skillet and cook for an additional 1-2 minutes, or until fragrant.

5. Stir in the dry green lentils, low-sodium vegetable broth, diced tomatoes (with juices), dried thyme, dried rosemary, paprika, salt, and pepper.

6. Bring the mixture to a boil, then reduce the heat to low. Cover and simmer for 25-30 minutes, or until the lentils are tender and the liquid is absorbed.

7. Transfer the lentil and vegetable mixture to a baking dish.

8. Spread the mashed potatoes over the top of the lentil mixture.

9. Bake in the preheated oven for 15-20 minutes, or until the mashed potatoes are lightly golden.

10. Garnish with chopped fresh parsley, if desired.

11. Serve the lentil and vegetable shepherd's pie hot.

Nutritional Value (per serving): Calories: 300 | Phosphorus: 200 mg | Sodium: 100 mg | Protein: 10 g | Carbohydrates: 45 g | Fats: 8 g | Potassium: 300 mg | Iron: 3 mg

Quinoa and Roasted Vegetable Buddha Bowl

Prep Time: 15 minutes | **Cook Time:** 25 minutes | **Total Time:** 40 minutes | **Per Serving:** 2 servings

Ingredients:

- 1 cup quinoa, rinsed
- 2 cups water
- 1 sweet potato, peeled and diced
- 1 red bell pepper, diced
- 1 zucchini, diced
- 1 tablespoon olive oil
- 1 teaspoon smoked paprika
- 1/2 teaspoon garlic powder
- Salt and pepper, to taste
- 2 cups baby spinach
- 1/2 cup hummus
- Lemon wedges, for serving

Instructions:

1. Preheat the oven to 400°F (200°C).
2. In a medium saucepan, bring the water to a boil. Add the quinoa, reduce the heat to low, cover, and simmer for 15 minutes, or until the quinoa is tender and the water has been absorbed. Remove from heat and let it sit, covered, for 5 minutes. Fluff with a fork.
3. While the quinoa is cooking, spread the diced sweet potato, red bell pepper, and zucchini on a baking sheet. Drizzle with olive oil and sprinkle with smoked paprika, garlic powder, salt, and pepper. Toss to coat.
4. Roast the vegetables in the preheated oven for 20-25 minutes, or until tender and lightly browned, stirring halfway through.
5. To assemble the Buddha bowls, divide the cooked quinoa and roasted vegetables between two bowls.
6. Add a handful of baby spinach to each bowl.
7. Top each bowl with a dollop of hummus.
8. Serve the quinoa and roasted vegetable Buddha bowls with lemon wedges on the side.

Nutritional Value (per serving): Calories: 350 | Phosphorus: 150 mg | Sodium: 100 mg | Protein: 10 g | Carbohydrates: 55 g | Fats: 10 g | Potassium: 300 mg | Iron: 3 mg

Tofu and Vegetable Stir-Fry with Brown Rice

Prep Time: 15 minutes | **Cook Time:** 20 minutes | **Total Time:** 35 minutes | **Per Serving:** 4 servings

Ingredients:

- 1 cup brown rice
- 2 cups water
- 1 tablespoon olive oil
- 1 block (14 ounces) of firm tofu, drained and cubed
- 2 cups broccoli florets
- 1 red bell pepper, sliced
- 1 carrot, sliced
- 1/2 cup low-sodium vegetable broth
- 2 tablespoons low-sodium soy sauce
- 1 tablespoon rice vinegar
- 1 tablespoon cornstarch
- 1 teaspoon grated ginger
- 2 cloves garlic, minced
- 2 green onions, sliced
- Sesame seeds, for garnish (optional)

Instructions:

1. In a medium saucepan, combine the brown rice and water. Bring to a boil, then reduce the heat to low, cover, and simmer for 45 minutes, or until the rice is tender and the water is absorbed. Remove from heat and let it sit, covered, for 5 minutes. Fluff with a fork.

2. While the rice is cooking, heat olive oil in a large skillet or wok over medium-high heat.

3. Add the cubed tofu to the skillet and cook until golden brown on all sides, about 5-7 minutes. Remove tofu from the skillet and set aside.

4. In the same skillet, add the broccoli, red bell pepper, and carrot. Cook, stirring occasionally, for 3-4 minutes, or until the vegetables are tender-crisp.

5. In a small bowl, whisk together the low-sodium vegetable broth, low-sodium soy sauce, rice vinegar, cornstarch, grated ginger, and minced garlic.

6. Return the tofu to the skillet and pour the sauce over the tofu and vegetables. Cook, stirring constantly, until the sauce has thickened, about 2-3 minutes.

7. Serve the tofu and vegetable stir-fry over cooked brown rice, garnished with sliced green onions and sesame seeds, if desired.

Nutritional Value (per serving): Calories: 300 | Phosphorus: 150 mg | Sodium: 100 mg | Protein: 15 g | Carbohydrates: 40 g | Fats: 10 g | Potassium: 300 mg | Iron: 3 mg

Eggplant and Chickpea Tagine with Couscous

Prep Time: 15 minutes | **Cook Time:** 30 minutes | **Total Time:** 45 minutes | **Per Serving:** 4 servings

Ingredients:

- 1 tablespoon olive oil
- 1 onion, diced
- 2 cloves garlic, minced
- 1 eggplant, diced
- 1 can (15 ounces) chickpeas, drained and rinsed
- 1 can (14 ounces) diced tomatoes
- 1 teaspoon ground cumin
- 1 teaspoon ground coriander
- 1/2 teaspoon ground cinnamon
- 1/2 teaspoon smoked paprika
- Salt and pepper, to taste
- 1 cup low-sodium vegetable broth
- 1 cup couscous
- Fresh cilantro, chopped, for garnish (optional)

Instructions:

1. Heat olive oil in a large skillet or tagine over medium heat.

2. Add the diced onion to the skillet. Cook, stirring occasionally, until the onion is soft and translucent, about 3-4 minutes.

3. Add the minced garlic to the skillet and cook for an additional 1-2 minutes, or until fragrant.

4. Add the diced eggplant to the skillet. Cook, stirring occasionally, until the eggplant is tender, about 5-7 minutes.

5. Stir in the drained and rinsed chickpeas, diced tomatoes (with juices), ground cumin, ground coriander, ground cinnamon, smoked paprika, salt, and pepper.

6. Pour the low-sodium vegetable broth into the skillet. Bring to a simmer and cook for 10-15 minutes, or until the flavors are well combined and the sauce has thickened slightly.

7. While the tagine is simmering, prepare the couscous according to the package instructions.

8. Serve the eggplant and chickpea tagine over cooked couscous.

9. Garnish with chopped fresh cilantro, if desired.

Nutritional Value (per serving): Calories: 300 | Phosphorus: 150 mg | Sodium: 100 mg | Protein: 10 g | Carbohydrates: 50 g | Fats: 8 g | Potassium: 300 mg | Iron: 3 mg

Mushroom and Lentil Bolognese with Whole Wheat Pasta

Prep Time: 15 minutes | **Cook Time:** 30 minutes | **Total Time:** 45 minutes | **Per Serving:** 4 servings

Ingredients:

- 1 tablespoon olive oil
- 1 onion, diced
- 2 cloves garlic, minced
- 8 ounces mushrooms, sliced
- 1 can (14 ounces) diced tomatoes
- 1 cup cooked brown lentils
- 1 teaspoon dried oregano
- 1 teaspoon dried basil
- 1/2 teaspoon dried thyme
- Salt and pepper, to taste
- 8 ounces whole wheat pasta
- Fresh parsley, chopped, for garnish (optional)

Instructions:

1. Heat olive oil in a large skillet over medium heat.
2. Add the diced onion to the skillet. Cook, stirring occasionally, until the onion is soft and translucent, about 3-4 minutes.
3. Add the minced garlic to the skillet and cook for an additional 1-2 minutes, or until fragrant.
4. Add the sliced mushrooms to the skillet. Cook, stirring occasionally, until the mushrooms are golden brown and tender, about 5-7 minutes.
5. Stir in the diced tomatoes (with juices), cooked brown lentils, dried oregano, dried basil, dried thyme, salt, and pepper.
6. Simmer the mushroom and lentil bolognese sauce for 10-15 minutes, or until the flavors are well combined and the sauce has thickened slightly.
7. While the sauce is simmering, cook the whole wheat pasta according to the package instructions.
8. Serve the mushroom and lentil bolognese sauce over cooked whole wheat pasta.
9. Garnish with chopped fresh parsley, if desired.

Nutritional Value (per serving): Calories: 350 | Phosphorus: 150 mg | Sodium: 100 mg | Protein: 15 g | Carbohydrates: 60 g | Fats: 5 g | Potassium: 300 mg | Iron: 4 mg

Cauliflower Steak with Chimichurri Sauce

Prep Time: 15 minutes | **Cook Time:** 25 minutes | **Total Time:** 40 minutes | **Per Serving:** 4 servings

Ingredients:

- 1 large head cauliflower, leaves removed
- 2 tablespoons olive oil
- Salt and pepper, to taste

Chimichurri Sauce:

- 1 cup fresh parsley, finely chopped
- 1/4 cup fresh cilantro, finely chopped
- 2 cloves garlic, minced
- 2 tablespoons red wine vinegar
- 1/4 cup olive oil
- 1/4 teaspoon red pepper flakes
- Salt and pepper, to taste

Instructions:

1. Preheat the oven to 425°F (220°C). Line a baking sheet with parchment paper.
2. Slice the cauliflower into 1-inch-thick steaks. Place the cauliflower steaks on the prepared baking sheet.
3. Brush both sides of the cauliflower steaks with olive oil. Season with salt and pepper.
4. Roast the cauliflower steaks in the preheated oven for 20-25 minutes, or until golden brown and tender, flipping halfway through.

Chimichurri Sauce:

1. In a small bowl, combine the chopped parsley, chopped cilantro, minced garlic, red wine vinegar, olive oil, red pepper flakes, salt, and pepper. Stir until well combined.

2. Taste and adjust seasoning, if necessary.

Assembly:

1. Place the roasted cauliflower steaks on a serving platter.

2. Drizzle the chimichurri sauce over the cauliflower steaks.

3. Serve immediately.

Nutritional Value (per serving): Calories: 150 | Phosphorus: 50 mg | Sodium: 50 mg | Protein: 5 g | Carbohydrates: 10 g | Fats: 10 g | Potassium: 300 mg | Iron: 2 mg

Spinach and White Bean Stuffed Bell Peppers

Prep Time: 15 minutes | **Cook Time:** 30 minutes | **Total Time:** 45 minutes | **Per Serving:** 4 servings

Ingredients:

- 4 bell peppers, halved and seeds removed
- 1 tablespoon olive oil
- 1 onion, diced
- 2 cloves garlic, minced
- 2 cups fresh spinach, chopped
- 1 can (15 ounces) white beans, drained and rinsed
- 1 cup cooked quinoa
- 1 teaspoon dried oregano
- 1 teaspoon dried basil
- Salt and pepper, to taste
- 1/4 cup shredded low-fat mozzarella cheese (optional)
- Fresh parsley, chopped, for garnish (optional)

Instructions:

1. Preheat the oven to 375°F (190°C). Lightly grease a baking dish.
2. Heat olive oil in a large skillet over medium heat.
3. Add the diced onion to the skillet. Cook, stirring occasionally, until the onion is soft and translucent, about 3-4 minutes.
4. Add the minced garlic to the skillet and cook for an additional 1-2 minutes, or until fragrant.
5. Add the chopped spinach to the skillet. Cook, stirring occasionally, until the spinach is wilted, about 2-3 minutes.
6. Stir in the white beans, cooked quinoa, dried oregano, dried basil, salt, and pepper. Cook for another 2-3 minutes, until heated through.
7. Spoon the spinach and white bean mixture into the halved bell peppers, dividing evenly.
8. Place the stuffed bell peppers in the prepared baking dish. If using, sprinkle the shredded low-fat mozzarella cheese over the stuffed peppers.

9. Cover the baking dish with aluminum foil and bake in the preheated oven for 25-30 minutes, or until the peppers are tender.

10. Garnish with chopped fresh parsley, if desired, before serving.

Nutritional Value (per serving): Calories: 200 | Phosphorus: 100 mg | Sodium: 50 mg | Protein: 10 g | Carbohydrates: 30 g | Fats: 5 g | Potassium: 300 mg | Iron: 3 mg

Coconut Curry Lentil Soup with Naan Bread

Prep Time: 15 minutes | **Cook Time:** 30 minutes | **Total Time:** 45 minutes | **Per Serving:** 4 servings

Ingredients:

- 1 tablespoon olive oil
- 1 onion, diced
- 2 cloves garlic, minced
- 1 tablespoon curry powder
- 1 teaspoon ground cumin
- 1/2 teaspoon ground turmeric
- 1 cup dried red lentils, rinsed and drained
- 4 cups low-sodium vegetable broth
- 1 can (14 ounces) light coconut milk
- 1 cup diced tomatoes
- 2 cups fresh spinach
- Salt and pepper, to taste
- Fresh cilantro, chopped, for garnish (optional)
- Naan bread, for serving

Instructions:

1. Heat olive oil in a large pot over medium heat.
2. Add the diced onion to the pot. Cook, stirring occasionally, until the onion is soft and translucent, about 3-4 minutes.
3. Add the minced garlic, curry powder, ground cumin, and ground turmeric to the pot. Cook, stirring constantly, for 1 minute, until fragrant.
4. Add the rinsed and drained red lentils, low-sodium vegetable broth, light coconut milk, and diced tomatoes to the pot. Bring to a simmer.
5. Simmer the soup, uncovered, for 20-25 minutes, or until the lentils are tender and the soup has thickened slightly.
6. Stir in the fresh spinach and cook for an additional 2-3 minutes, until the spinach is wilted.
7. Season the soup with salt and pepper, to taste.
8. Ladle the coconut curry lentil soup into bowls. Garnish with chopped fresh cilantro, if desired.
9. Serve the soup with warm naan bread on the side.

Nutritional Value (per serving): Calories: 250 | Phosphorus: 150 mg | Sodium: 100 mg | Protein: 10 g | Carbohydrates: 30 g | Fats: 8 g | Potassium: 300 mg | Iron: 3 mg

Practical Tips and Resources

Cooking Techniques for CKD

Low-Sodium Cooking Methods

1. Steaming:

- Description: Steaming is a gentle cooking method that helps retain nutrients without the need for added fats or oils.
- How to Use: Steam vegetables, fish, and even grains like quinoa.
- Benefits: Preserve the natural flavors and textures of foods while minimizing the need for added sodium.

2. Boiling:

- Description: Boiling is a simple method that works well for cooking pasta, grains, and vegetables.
- How to Use: Use unsalted water or low-sodium broth for boiling.
- Benefits: An easy and quick cooking method that requires minimal added ingredients.

3. Poaching:

- Description: Poaching involves gently simmering food in liquid, such as water or broth, at a low temperature.
- How to Use: Ideal for cooking delicate foods like fish and chicken breasts.
- Benefits: Preserve the moisture and tenderness of foods without the need for added fats.

4. Grilling/Broiling:

- Description: Grilling or broiling adds flavor without the need for added fats.
- How to Use: Be cautious with marinades and sauces, as they can often be high in sodium.
- Benefits: Creates delicious caramelization and adds smoky flavor to foods.

Flavor Enhancing without Salt

1. **Herbs and Spices:**

    - Description: Use a variety of herbs and spices to add flavor to your dishes without adding salt.

    - How to Use: Experiment with basil, oregano, thyme, rosemary, cumin, paprika, and more to enhance the taste of your meals.

    - Benefits: Adds depth and complexity to dishes without increasing sodium intake.

2. **Citrus:**

    - Description: Squeeze fresh lemon, lime, or orange juice over your dishes to add a burst of citrus flavor.

    - How to Use: Use citrus juice as a finishing touch for meats, seafood, salads, and vegetables.

    - Benefits: Provides acidity and brightness to dishes without the need for salt.

3. **Vinegar:**

    - Description: Balsamic vinegar, apple cider vinegar, and rice vinegar can add tanginess to your meals without the need for salt.

    - How to Use: Use as a marinade, salad dressing ingredient, or as a flavor enhancer for cooked dishes.

    - Benefits: Adds complexity and depth of flavor to dishes while reducing the need for salt.

4. **Aromatics:**

    - Description: Onions, garlic, shallots, and leeks can add depth of flavor to your dishes without adding extra sodium.

    - How to Use: Sauté aromatics in a small amount of oil as a flavorful base for soups, stews, and sauces.

    - Benefits: Enhances the savory profile of dishes and adds complexity to the overall flavor.

Cooking for Texture and Variety

1. Roasting:

- Description: Roasting vegetables and meats can bring out their natural sweetness and create delicious caramelization.
- How to Use: Use a light coating of olive oil and your favorite herbs and spices to enhance flavor.
- Benefits: Adds depth of flavor and texture to dishes without the need for added fats.

2. Stir-Frying:

- Description: Stir-frying is a quick cooking method that works well for vegetables, lean meats, and tofu.
- How to Use: Use a non-stick pan and a small amount of oil for a healthy cooking option.
- Benefits: Preserve the natural crunch and color of vegetables while cooking them quickly to retain nutrients.

3. Baking:

- Description: Baking is a healthy cooking method that doesn't require added fats.
- How to Use: Use it for preparing casseroles, baked fish, and roasted vegetables.
- Benefits: Provides even cooking and allows flavors to meld together while keeping dishes moist and flavorful.

4. Sautéing:

- Description: Sautéing quickly cooks food in a small amount of oil over medium-high heat.
- How to Use: Ideal for cooking vegetables, lean meats, and seafood.
- Benefits: Preserve the natural texture and flavor of foods while cooking them quickly and efficiently.

Conclusion

Living with chronic kidney disease (CKD) presents unique challenges, particularly when it comes to maintaining a kidney-friendly diet. However, with the right knowledge and resources, it is possible to enjoy delicious and satisfying meals while supporting kidney health.

In this comprehensive guide, we have explored various aspects of managing CKD through diet, including understanding the stages of CKD, nutritional needs, and restrictions, building a CKD-friendly pantry, and practical tips for meal planning and shopping.

We have provided a wide range of kidney-friendly recipes for every meal of the day, ensuring that you have plenty of options to choose from while adhering to low potassium, low sodium, and low phosphorus dietary restrictions. From hearty breakfasts to flavorful dinners, satisfying snacks, and refreshing beverages, each recipe has been carefully crafted to provide maximum flavor and nutrition without compromising kidney health.

By incorporating low-sodium cooking methods, flavor-enhancing techniques without salt, and cooking for texture and variety, you can create delicious meals that support your overall health and well-being.

With the knowledge and recipes provided in this guide, we hope you feel empowered to take control of your kidney health and enjoy a diverse and flavorful diet that nourishes your body and soul.

Here's to delicious, kidney-friendly eating and a healthier, happier you!

www.ingramcontent.com/pod-product-compliance
Lightning Source LLC
Chambersburg PA
CBHW082207220526
45470CB00010B/3071